JRCALC Clinical Guidelines 1

POC

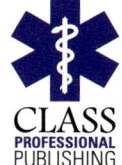

CLASS PROFESSIONAL PUBLISHING

Disclaimer

This Pocket Book has been produced by the Joint Royal Colleges Ambulance Liaison Comittee (JRCALC) and is based on the JRCALC Clinical Guidelines. The complete guidelines are available on iCPG and JRCALC Plus, the JRCALC apps, and published in print format as the JRCALC Clinical Guidelines. **Updates to guidelines and medicines dosages are published on the JRCALC apps, iCPG and JRCALC Plus, as required. The JRCALC apps contain the complete and most current information.**

The Pocket Book is intended to be used by clinicians working in the ambulance service as an aide-memoire and to confirm safe therapeutic drug dosages prior to administration. It also contains treatment algorithms and management plans that are intended to be used as a quick reference guide only. As such it is designed to be used in conjunction with the JRCALC apps and the JRCALC Clinical Guidelines 2019 which contain the full text that cannot be reproduced in this Pocket Book.

The Association of Ambulance Chief Executives and the Joint Royal Colleges Ambulance Liaison Committee have made every effort to ensure that the information, tables, drawings and diagrams contained in these guidelines are accurate at the time of publication. However, the guidelines are advisory and have been developed to assist healthcare professionals, and patients, to make decisions about the management of the patient's health, including treatments. This advice is intended to support the decision making process and is not a substitute for sound clinical judgement. The guidelines cannot always contain all the information necessary for determining appropriate care and cannot address all individual situations; therefore, individuals using these guidelines must ensure they have the appropriate knowledge and skills to enable suitable interpretation.

The Association of Ambulance Chief Executives and the Joint Royal Colleges Ambulance Liaison Committee do not guarantee, and accept no legal liability of whatever nature arising from or connected to, the accuracy, reliability, currency or completeness of the content of these guidelines. Users of these guidelines must always be aware that such innovations or alterations after the date of publication may not be incorporated in the content. As part of its commitment to defining national standards, JRCALC will periodically issue updates to the content and users should ensure that they are using the most up to date version of the guidelines. These updates can be found on the JRCALC apps and aace.org.uk. Please note however that the Association of Ambulance Chief Executives assumes no responsibility whatsoever for the content of external resources.

Although some modification of the guidelines may be required by individual ambulance services, and approved by the relevant local clinical committees, to ensure they respond to the health requirements of the local community, the majority of the guidance is universally applicable to NHS ambulance services. Modification of the guidelines may also occur when undertaking research sanctioned by a research committee.

Whilst these guidelines cover a range of paramedic treatments available across the UK they will also provide a valuable tool for a range of care providers. Many of the assessment skills and general principles will remain the same. All clinical staff must practice with

© Association of Ambulance Chief Executives (AACE) 2021

All rights reserved. Without limiting the rights under copyright reserved above, no part of this publication may be reproduced, stored in or introduced into a retrieval system, or transmitted, in any form or by any means (electronic, mechanical, photocopying, recording or otherwise) without the prior written permission of the publisher of this book.

The information presented in this book is accurate and current to the best of the authors' knowledge. The authors and publisher, however, make no guarantee as to, and assume no responsibility for, the correctness, sufficiency or completeness of such information or recommendation.

Printing history
First edition published 2013, reprinted 2013, 2015.
2016 edition published 2016, reprinted 2016.
2017 edition published 2017, reprinted 2017, 2018.
2019 edition published 2019.
This edition published 2021.

The authors and publisher welcome feedback from the users of this book. Please contact the publisher:
Class Professional Publishing,
The Exchange, Express Park, Bristol Road, Bridgwater TA6 4RR
Telephone: 01278 427 800 Email: cservs@class.co.uk
www.classprofessional.co.uk

Class Professional Publishing is an imprint of Class Publishing Ltd

A CIP catalogue record for this book is available from the British Library
ISBN 978 1 85959 902 0

Designed and typeset by PageMajik

Printed and bound in Italy by L.E.G.O.

This edition:
JRCALC Clinical Guidelines 2021 Pocket Book
ISBN 978 1 85959 902 0 (print edition)

Also available:
JRCALC Clinical Guidelines 2021 Pocket Book
ISBN 9781859599037 (eBook)

RESUSCITATION   1

Basic Life Support (Adult)   **2**
Airway: Assessment and
  Management overview   **3**
Advanced Life Support (Adult)   **4**
Return of Spontaneous
  Circulation   **6**
UK Risk Assessment for
  Submersion   **8**
Implantable Cardioverter
  Defibrillator   **9**
Foreign Body Airway
  Obstruction (Adult)   **10**

PAEDIATRICS   11

Basic Life Support (Child)   **12**
Foreign Body Airway
  Obstruction (Child)   **13**
Advanced Life Support (Child)   **14**
Death of a Child   **16**
The FLACC Scale   **17**
GREEN: NICE 'Traffic Lights'
  Clinical Assessment Tool
  for Febrile Ilness in Children   **18**
AMBER: NICE 'Traffic Lights'
  Clinical Assessment Tool
  for Febrile Illness in Children   **19**
RED: NICE 'Traffic Lights' Clinical
  Assessment Tool for Febrile
  Illness in Children   **20**

Modified Taussig Croup Score   **21**
Meningococcal Meningitis
  and Septicaemia   **22**
Peak Expiratory Flow Chart   **23**
Convulsions (Children)   **24**
Trauma Emergencies
  Overview (Children)   **26**

GENERAL   29

Pain Management in Adults   **30**
Pain Assessment Model   **31**
Glasgow Coma Scale   **32**
National Early Warning
  Score (NEWS2)   **33**
IPAP Suicide Risk Assessment
  Tool   **34**
IPAP Suggested Actions   **35**
Mental Capacity Assessment
  in Brief   **36**

MEDICAL   37

Adult Bradycardia Algorithm   **38**
Adult Tachycardia
  (With Pulse)   **39**
Heart Failure   **40**
Pulmonary Embolism   **41**
Asthma   **42**
Asthma Features of Severity   **43**
Asthma Peak Flow Charts   **44**
Chronic Obstructive Pulmonary
  Disease   **45**

Convulsions (Adults)	**46**
Glycaemic Emergencies (Adults)	**48**
Allergic Reactions including Anaphylaxis	**50**
Sickle Cell Crisis	**51**

🟥 TRAUMA **53**

Trauma – ATMIST	**54**
Trauma Survey	**55**
Trauma Emergencies Overview (Adults)	**56**
Spinal Injury and Spinal Cord Injury	**58**

🟧 SPECIAL SITUATIONS **61**

METHANE Report Format	**62**
Triage Sieve	**63**
Specialist Capabilities	**64**

🟪 MATERNITY **67**

Maternity Care	**68**
Breech Birth	**69**
Cord Prolapse	**70**
Eclampsia	**71**
Newborn Life Support	**72**
Normal Birth	**73**
Post-partum Haemorrhage	**74**
Shoulder Dystocia	**75**

🟧 MEDICINES **77**

Medicines: Best Practice Checklist	**78**
Activated Charcoal	**79**
Adrenaline 1 milligram in 10 ml (1 in 10,000)	**83**
Adrenaline 1 milligram in 1 ml (1 in 1,000)	**85**
Amiodarone Hydrochloride	**87**
Aspirin	**89**
Atropine Sulfate	**91**
Benzylpenicillin Sodium	**95**
Chlorphenamine	**97**
Clopidogrel	**100**
Dexamethasone	**103**
Diazepam	**109**
Furosemide	**114**
Glucagon	**116**
Glucose 10%	**119**
Glucose 40% Oral Gel	**122**
Glyceryl Trinitrate (GTN)	**124**
Heparin (Unfractionated)	**128**
Hydrocortisone	**131**
Ibuprofen	**135**
Ipratropium Bromide	**138**
Metoclopramide Hydrochloride	**141**
Midazolam	**143**
Misoprostol	**146**

Morphine Sulfate	**149**	6 MONTHS	**266**
Naloxone Hydrochloride	**163**	9 MONTHS	**272**
Nitrous Oxide (Entonox®)	**169**	12 MONTHS	**278**
Ondansetron	**172**	18 MONTHS	**284**
Oxygen	**175**	2 YEARS	**290**
Paracetamol	**190**	3 YEARS	**298**
Salbutamol	**201**	4 YEARS	**304**
Sodium Chloride 0.9%	**205**	5 YEARS	**310**
Sodium Lactate Compound	**220**	6 YEARS	**316**
Syntometrine	**233**	7 YEARS	**322**
Tenecteplase	**235**	8 YEARS	**328**
Tranexamic Acid	**239**	9 YEARS	**334**
		10 YEARS	**340**
PAGE FOR AGE	**245**	11 YEARS	**346**
BIRTH	**246**		
1 MONTH	**252**		
3 MONTHS	**260**		

RESUSCITATION

RESUS

Basic Life Support (Adult)

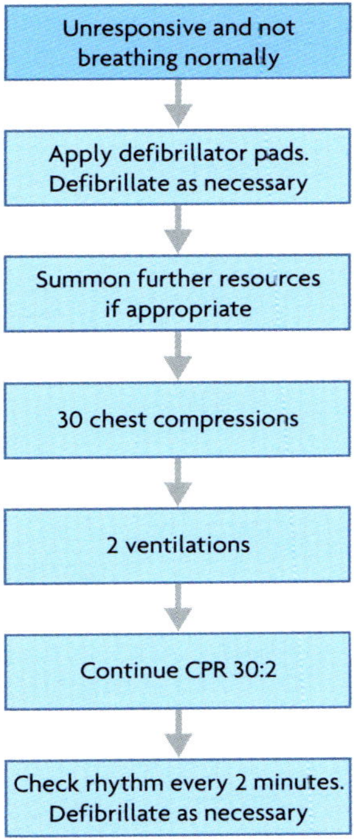

Unresponsive and not
breathing normally

↓

Apply defibrillator pads.
Defibrillate as necessary

↓

Summon further resources
if appropriate

↓

30 chest compressions

↓

2 ventilations

↓

Continue CPR 30:2

↓

Check rhythm every 2 minutes.
Defibrillate as necessary

Reproduced with permission from the Resuscitation Council (UK)
Guidelines 2015 (www.resus.org.uk)
Refer to **Paediatrics** for the child guideline

Airway
Breathing assessment and management overview

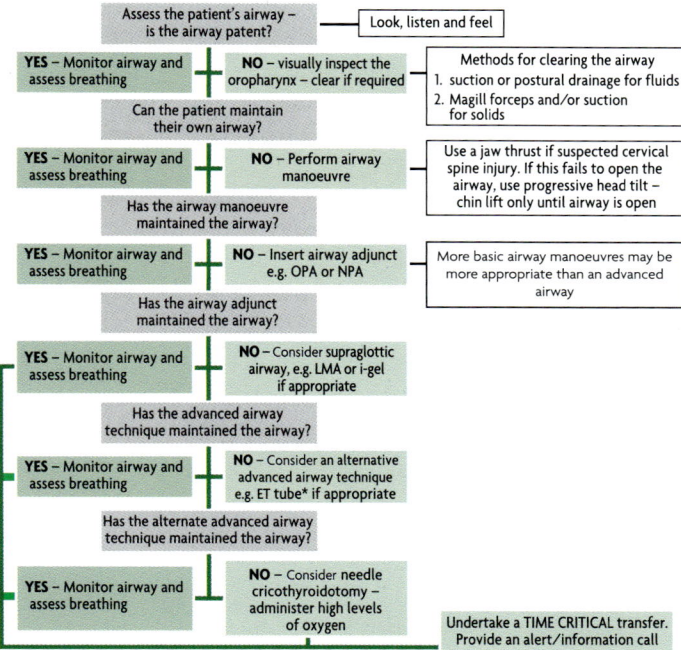

*Endotracheal intubation must only be performed when waveform capnography is available.

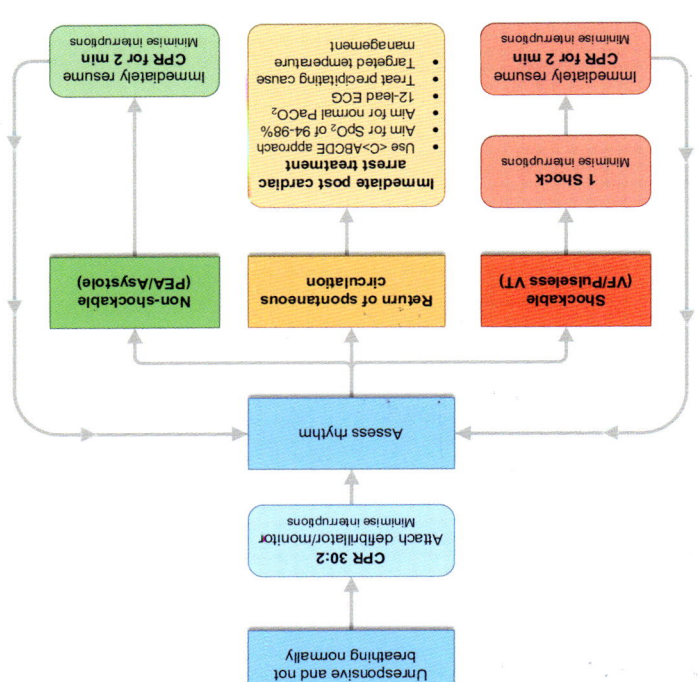

Advanced Life Support (Adult)

During CPR
- Ensure high quality chest compressions
- Minimise interruptions to compressions
- Give oxygen
- Use waveform capnography
- Continuous compressions when advanced airway in place
- Vascular access (intravenous or intraosseous)
- Give adrenaline every 3-5 min
- Give amiodarone after 3 shocks, consider half dose after 5th shock

Treat Reversible Causes
- Hypoxia
- Hypovolaemia
- Hypo-/hyperkalaemia/metabolic
- Hypothermia
- Thrombosis - coronary or pulmonary
- Tension pneumothorax
- Tamponade – cardiac
- Toxins

Consider
- Ultrasound imaging
- Mechanical chest compressions to facilitate transfer/treatment
- Coronary angiography and percutaneous coronary intervention
- Extracorporeal CPR

Reproduced with permission from the Resuscitation Council (UK) Guidelines 2015 algorithm (www.resus.org.uk).

1°: DRsABCDE → primary assessment

2°: SAMPLER → secondary survey.

- Signs & Symptoms
- Allergies
- Medication
- Past medical history
- last oral intake
- events leading to
- reccomendation

RESUS

Return of Spontaneous Circulation

Prepare for Transfer
a. Early recurrence of VF is common; ensure appropriate ongoing monitoring through defibrillator pads.
b. Transfer the patient directly to the nearest appropriate hospital in accordance with local pathways.
c. Provide an ATMIST pre-alert call to the receiving facility.

Airway & Breathing
a. Ensure an effective airway; consider enhanced support
b. Record and maintain oxygen saturations of 94–98%, refer to Oxygen.
c. Monitor waveform capnography.
d. Ventilate lungs to normocarbia (4.6–6.0 kPa)

Circulation
a. Record blood pressure and aim for SBP > 90 mmHg.
b. First: Fluid (crystalloid) – restore normovolaemia. Refer to Intravascular Fluid in Adults and Intravascular Fluid in Children.
c. Second: Consider vasopressor/inotrope to maintain SBP unresponsive to fluid resuscitation as per local guideline (if this exists), e.g. adrenaline.
d. In the event of symptomatic bradycardia, atropine should be administered, refer to Atropine.

Return of Spontaneous Circulation

ECG
Perform a 12-lead ECG

Temperature
a. Measure temperature.
b. Patients post-ROSC should be allowed to cool passively.

BM
Measure and record blood glucose for hypo/hyperglycaemia, refer to Glycaemic Emergencies in Adults and Children.

Other
a. Consider the provision of analgesia (small dose opiates or IV Paracetamol) for the management of pain
b. Seizures that do not self-terminate within five minutes may be treated with a benzodiazepine, refer to Diazepam.
c. Combative patients may benefit from anaesthetic management or sedation. Consider enhanced care.

UK Risk Assessment for Submersion

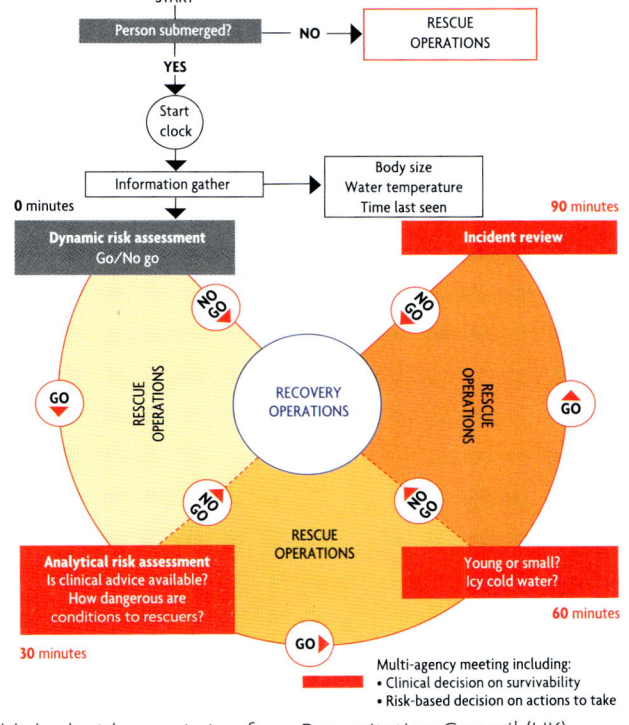

Republished with permission from Resuscitation Council (UK).

Implantable Cardioverter Defibrillator

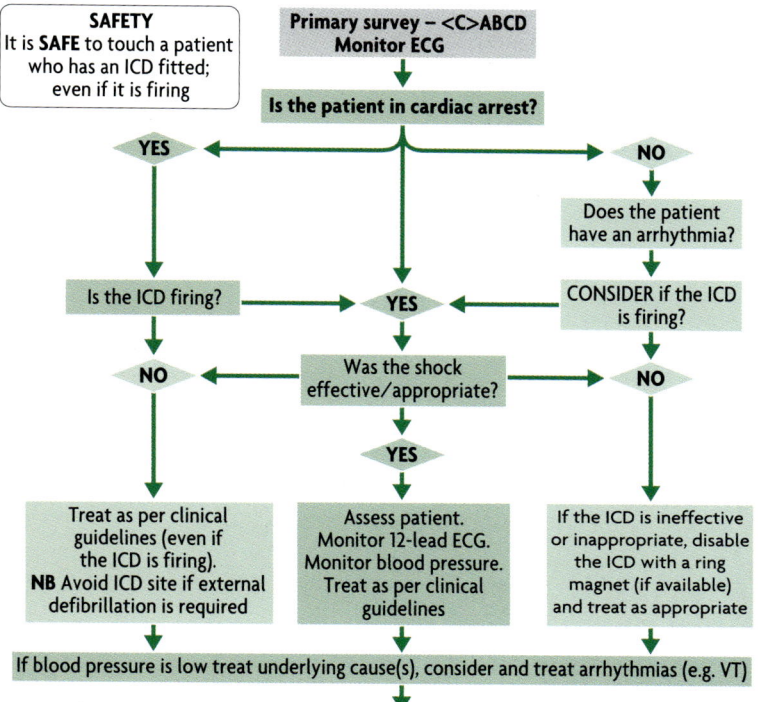

RESUS

Foreign Body Airway Obstruction (Adult)

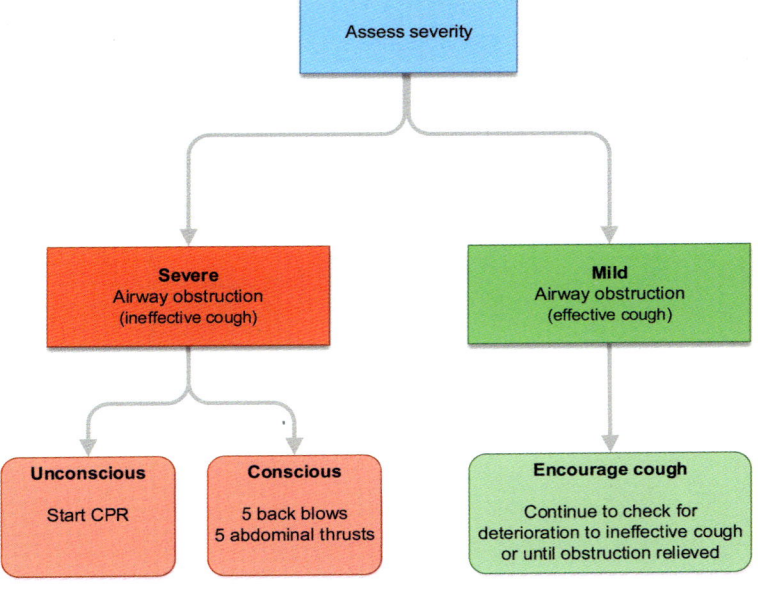

Reproduced with permission from the Resuscitation Council (UK) Guidelines 2015 algorithm (www.resus.org.uk)

PAEDIATRICS

PAED

Basic Life Support (Child)

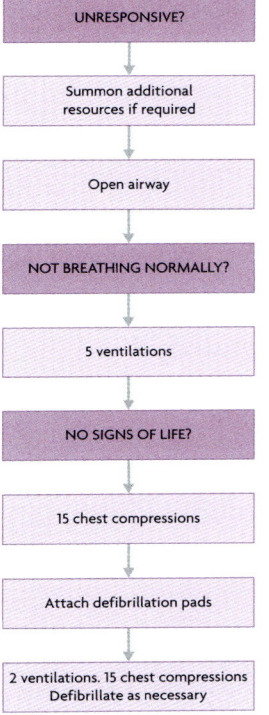

Reproduced with permission from the Resuscitation Council (UK)
Guidelines 2015 algorithm (www.resus.org.uk)

Foreign Body Airway Obstruction (Child)

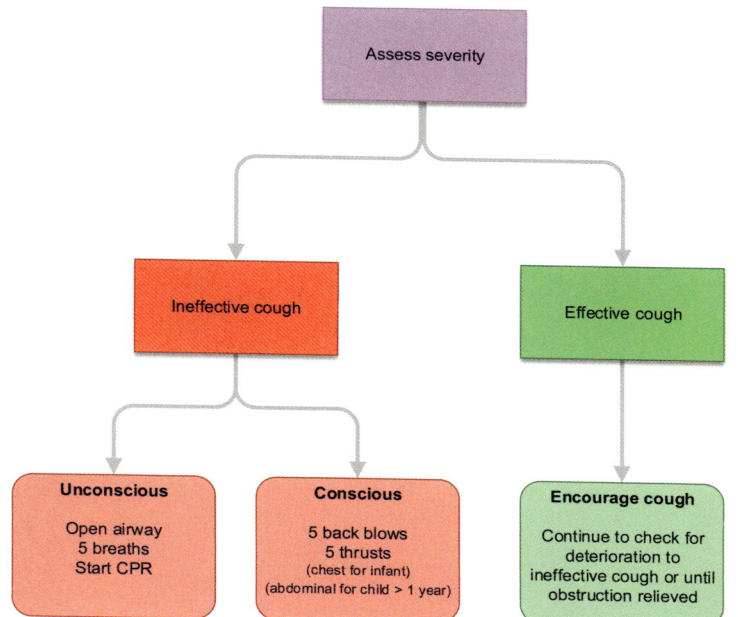

Reproduced with permission from the Resuscitation Council (UK) Guidelines 2015 algorithm (www.resus.org.uk)

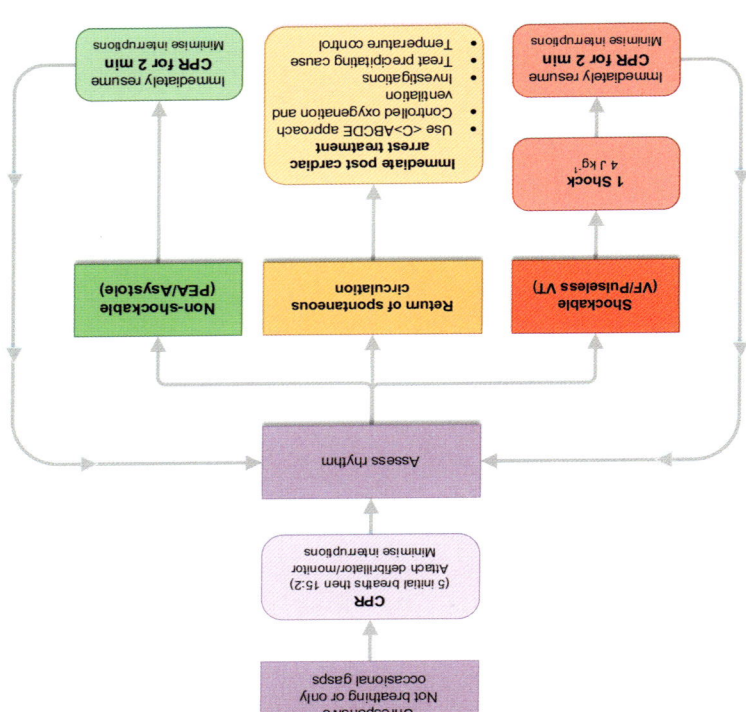

Advanced Life Support (Child)

During CPR
- Ensure high-quality CPR: rate, depth, recoil
- Plan actions before interrupting CPR
- Give oxygen
- Vascular access (intravenous, intraosseous)
- Give adrenaline every 3-5 min
- Consider advanced airway and capnography
- Continuous chest compressions when advanced airway in place
- Correct reversible causes
- Consider amiodarone after 3 and 5 shocks

Reversible Causes
- Hypoxia
- Hypovolaemia
- Hyper/hypokalaemia, metabolic
- Hypothermia

- Thrombosis (coronary or pulmonary)
- Tension pneumothorax
- Tamponade (cardiac)
- Toxic/therapeutic disturbances

Reproduced with permission from the Resuscitation Council (UK) Guidelines 2015 (www.resus.org.uk)

PAED

Death of a Child

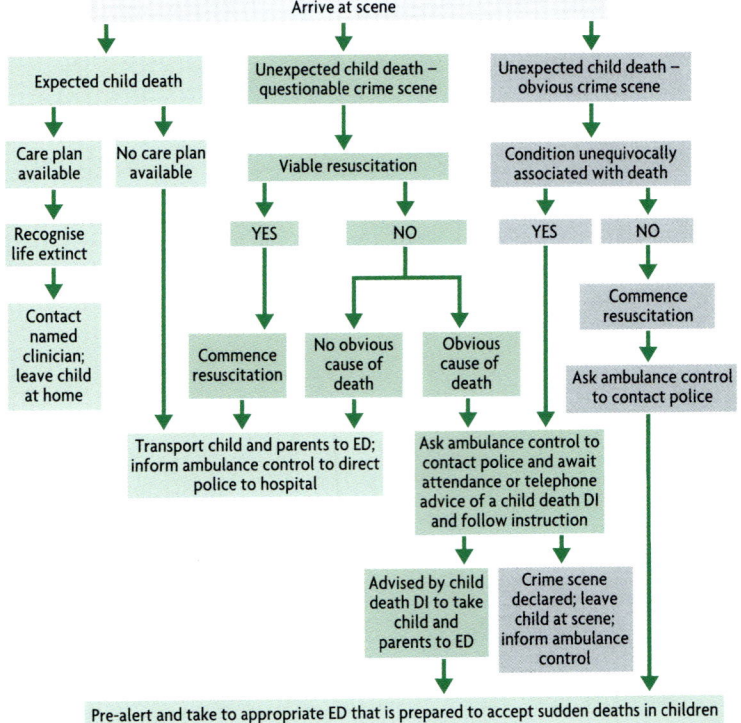

The FLACC Scale

The **Face, Legs, Activity, Cry, Consolability scale** or **FLACC scale** is a measurement used to assess pain for children up to the age of 7 years or individuals who are unable to communicate their pain. The scale is scored on a range of 0–10 with 0 representing no pain. The scale has five criteria which are each assigned a score of 0, 1 or 2.

Criteria	Score - 0	Score - 1	Score - 2
Face	No particular expression or smile	Occasional grimace or frown, withdrawn, uninterested	Frequent to constant quivering chin, clenched jaw
Legs	Normal position or relaxed	Uneasy, restless, tense	Kicking, or legs drawn up
Activity	Lying quietly, normal position, moves easily	Squirming, shifting back and forth, tense	Arched, rigid or jerking
Cry	No cry (awake or asleep)	Moans or whimpers, occasional complaint	Crying steadily, screams or sobs, frequent complaints
Consolability	Content, relaxed	Reassured by occasional touching, hugging or being talked to, distractible	Difficult to console or comfort

Refer also to the Wong–Baker Faces Pain Rating Scale, available at: wongbakerfaces.org

PAED

GREEN: NICE 'Traffic Lights' Clinical Assessment Tool for Febrile Illness in Children

Colour (of skin, lips or tongue)	Normal colour
Activity	Responds normally to social cues Content/smiles Stays awake or awakens quickly Strong normal cry/not crying
Circulation and hydration	Normal skin and eyes Moist mucous membranes
Other	None of the amber or red symptoms or signs

AMBER: NICE 'Traffic Lights' Clinical Assessment Tool for Febrile Illness in Children

Colour (of skin, lips or tongue)	Pallor reported by parent/carer
Activity	Not responding normally to social cues No smile Wakes only with prolonged stimulation Decreased activity
Respiratory	Nasal flaring Tachypnoea: • RR >50 breaths/min age 6–12 months • RR >40 breaths/min age >12 months O_2 sats ≤ 95% in air Crackles in the chest
Circulation and hydration	Tachycardia: • >160 beats/minute, age <12 months • >150 beats/minute, age 12–24 months • >140 beats/minute, age 2–5 years Dry mucous membranes Poor feeding in infants Capillary Refill Time (CRT) ≥3 seconds ↓Urinary output
Other	Age 3–6 months, temperature ≥39°C Fever for ≥5 days Swelling of a limb or joint Non-weight bearing limb/not using an extremity Rigors

PAED

RED: NICE 'Traffic Lights' Clinical Assessment Tool for Febrile Illness in Children

Colour (of skin, lips or tongue)	Pale/mottled/ashen/blue
Activity	No response to social cues Appears ill to a healthcare professional Does not wake, or if roused, does not stay awake Weak/high pitched/continuous cry
Respiratory	Grunting Tachypnoea: RR >60 breaths/min Moderate or severe chest indrawing
Circulation and hydration	Reduced skin turgor
Other	Age <3 months, temp ≥38°C (Some vaccinations have been found to induce fever in children aged under 3 months) Non-blanching rash Bulging fontanelle Neck stiffness Status epilepticus Focal seizures Focal neurological signs

Modified Taussig Croup Score

		Score*
Stridor	None	0
	Only on crying, exertion	1
	At rest	2
	Severe (biphasic)	3
Recession	None	0
	Only on crying, exertion	1
	At rest	2
	Severe (biphasic)	3

* Mild: 1–2; Moderate: 3–4; Severe: 5–6

PAED

Meningococcal Meningitis and Septicaemia

Management algorithm for patients with suspected meningococcal disease.

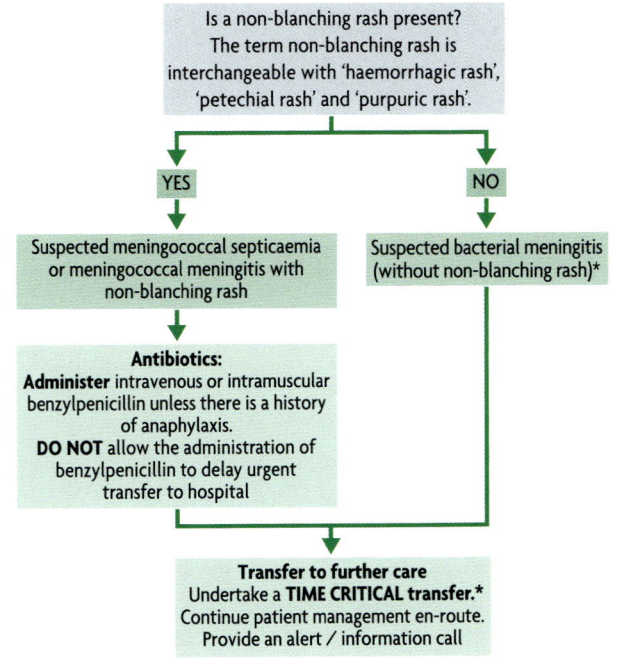

Is a non-blanching rash present?
The term non-blanching rash is interchangeable with 'haemorrhagic rash', 'petechial rash' and 'purpuric rash'.

YES

NO

Suspected meningococcal septicaemia or meningococcal meningitis with non-blanching rash

Suspected bacterial meningitis (without non-blanching rash)*

Antibiotics:
Administer intravenous or intramuscular benzylpenicillin unless there is a history of anaphylaxis.
DO NOT allow the administration of benzylpenicillin to delay urgent transfer to hospital

Transfer to further care
Undertake a **TIME CRITICAL** transfer.*
Continue patient management en-route.
Provide an alert / information call

* If bacterial meningitis is suspected and urgent transfer is not possible, administer antibiotics even in the absence of a non-blanching rash.

Peak Expiratory Flow Chart

Height (m)	Height (ft)	Predicted EU PEFR (L/min)
0.85	2'9"	87
0.90	2'11"	95
0.95	3'1"	104
1.00	3'3"	115
1.05	3'5"	127
1.10	3'7"	141
1.15	3'9"	157
1.20	3'11"	174
1.25	4'1"	192
1.30	4'3"	212
1.35	4'5"	233
1.40	4'7"	254
1.45	4'9"	276
1.50	4'11"	299
1.55	5'1"	323
1.60	5'3"	346
1.65	5'5"	370
1.70	5'7"	393

PAED

Convulsions (Children)

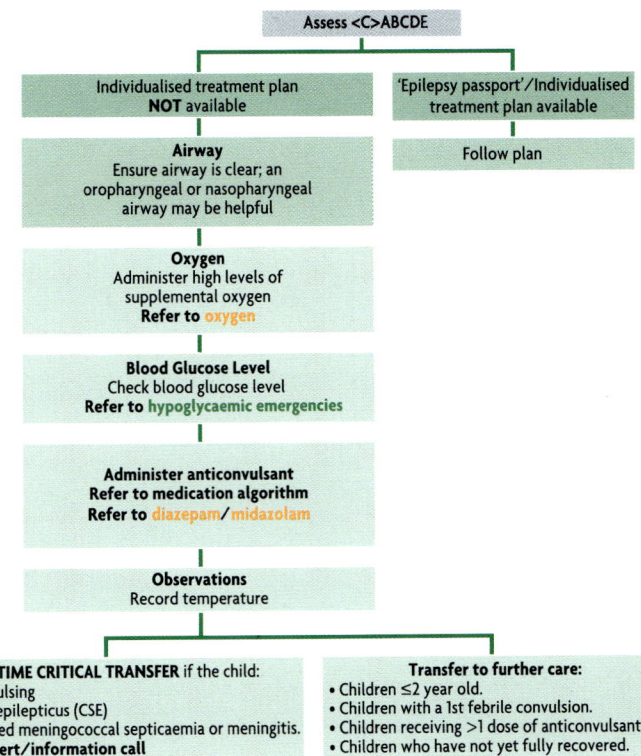

Assess <C>ABCDE

Individualised treatment plan NOT available

'Epilepsy passport'/Individualised treatment plan available

Follow plan

Airway
Ensure airway is clear; an oropharyngeal or nasopharyngeal airway may be helpful

Oxygen
Administer high levels of supplemental oxygen
Refer to oxygen

Blood Glucose Level
Check blood glucose level
Refer to hypoglycaemic emergencies

Administer anticonvulsant
Refer to medication algorithm
Refer to diazepam/midazolam

Observations
Record temperature

Undertake a **TIME CRITICAL TRANSFER** if the child:
• is still convulsing
• is in status epilepticus (CSE)
• has suspected meningococcal septicaemia or meningitis.
Provide an **alert/information call**

Transfer to further care:
• Children ≤2 year old.
• Children with a 1st febrile convulsion.
• Children receiving >1 dose of anticonvulsant.
• Children who have not yet fully recovered.

Convulsions (Children)

Medication algorithm for convulsions in children.

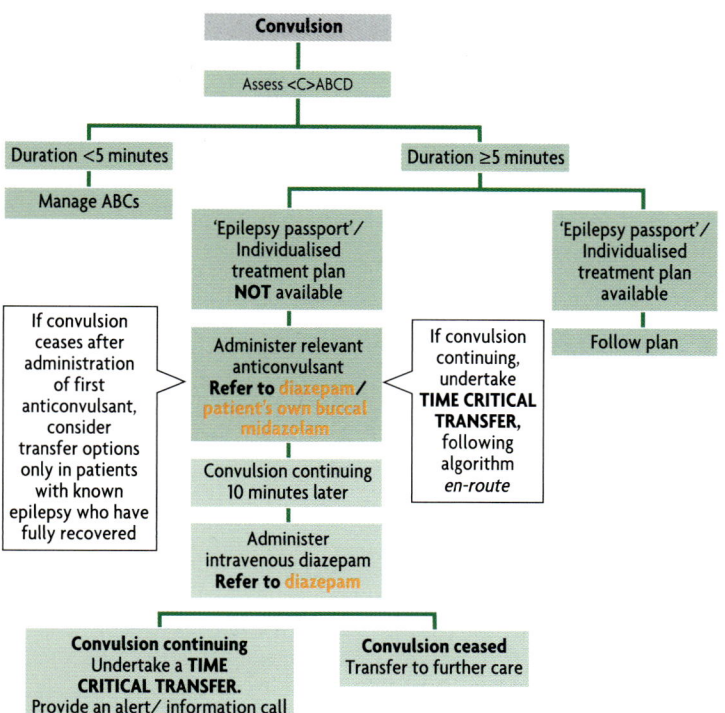

PAED

Trauma Emergencies Overview (Children)

The management of haemorrhage algorithm.

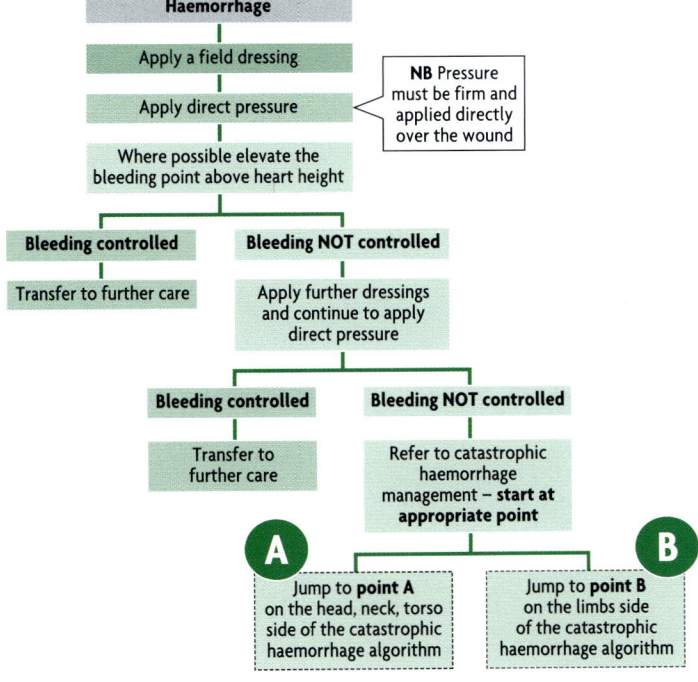

Trauma Emergencies Overview (Children)

The management of catastrophic haemorrhage algorithm.

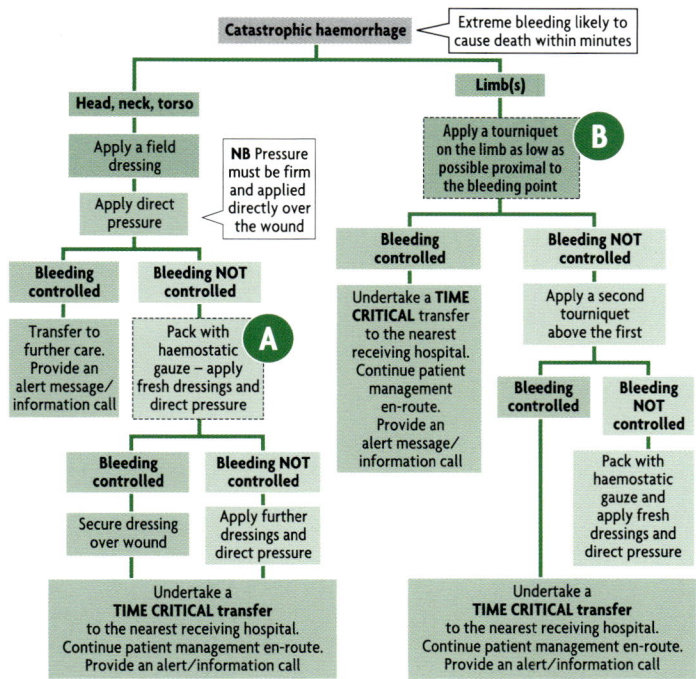

GENERAL

GENERAL

Pain Management in Adults

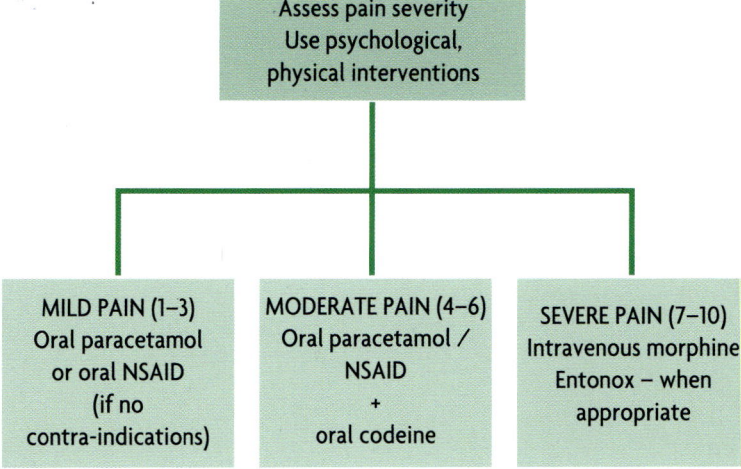

P = provocation: what provokes?
Q = quality: Sharp? dull?

Pain Assessment Model

S	Site	Where exactly is the pain?
O	Onset	What were they doing when the pain started?
C	Character	What does the pain feel like?
R	Radiates	Does the pain go anywhere else?
A	Associated symptoms	e.g. nausea/vomiting
T	Time/duration	How long have they had the pain?
E	Exacerbating/relieving factors	Does anything make the pain better or worse?
S	Severity	Obtain an initial pain score

O P Q R S T A

GENERAL

Glasgow Coma Scale

Category	Element	Score
Eyes Opening	Spontaneously	4
	To speech	3
	To pain	2
	None	1
Verbal Response	Orientated	5
	Confused	4
	Inappropriate words	3
	Incomprehensible sounds	2
	No verbal response	1
Motor Response	Obeys commands	6
	Localises pain	5
	Withdraws from pain	4
	Abnormal flexion	3
	Extensor response	2
	No response to pain	1

National Early Warning Score (NEWS2)

Physiological parameter	3	2	1	0	1	2	3
Respiration rate (per minute)	≤8		9–11	12–20		21–24	≥25
SpO$_2$ Scale 1 (%)	≤91	92–93	94–95	≥96			
SpO$_2$ Scale 2 (%)	≤83	84–85	86–87	88–92 ≥93 on air	93–94 on oxygen	95–96 on oxygen	≥97 on oxygen
Air or oxygen?		Oxygen		Air			
Systolic blood pressure (mmHg)	≤90	91–100	101–110	111–219			≥220
Pulse (per minute)	≤40		41–50	51–90	91–110	111–130	≥131
Consciousness				Alert			CVPU
Temperature (°C)	≤35.0		35.1–36.0	36.1–38.0	38.1–39.0	≥39.1	

NEWS2 chart. Reproduced from: Royal College of Physicians. National Early Warning Score (NEWS) 2:
Standardising the assessment of acute-illness severity in the NHS. Updated report of a working party. London: RCP, 2017.
Available at: https://www.rcplondon.ac.uk/projects/outputs/national-early-warning-score-news-2

GENERAL

IPAP Suicide Risk Assessment Tool

<u>NOTE</u>: **Always** consider the below in conjunction with other known risk factors such as age, gender, employment status and significant life events (e.g. relationship breakdown/divorce, bereavement, child birth).

INTENT	Is the patient experiencing suicidal thoughts now? Explore: Content, frequency and intrusiveness.
PLAN	Has the patient made any plans? ● What are they? ● Are they practical? ● Have they been rehearsed? ● Is there access to the means, and are the means readily available?
ACTION	Has any action been taken, present or past? **Present:** Has the patient carried out any acts in anticipation of death (e.g. putting their affairs in order, hoarding medication?) **Past:** History of mental illness, previous suicide attempt, self-harm or substance misuse = higher risk of completing suicide.
PROTECTIVE MEASURES (**LACK** of these increases the risk)	What support does the patient have access to now? Consider: Family, friends and health and social care services.

IPAP Suggested Actions

No thoughts of killing self.	Routine appointment with GP. Ring Samaritans on 116 123 if the patient would like to speak to someone. This is a free 24/7 number. If symptoms worsen, contact emergency care.
Some/vague thoughts. No plan. Thoughts and/or vague plan.	Patient must be seen by a mental health practitioner. Consider: ● Mental Health Pathways, access to mental health services, crisis teams or crisis cafes etc. ● Contact the GP for an urgent appointment. ● GP Triage or similar.
Repeated thoughts and/or specific plan. Access to means. Persistent thoughts of killing self.	Patient must be seen by a mental health specialist practitioner as soon as possible. If known to local mental health services contact the Care Co-ordinator. If not known, contact local urgent access services or GP. If none available take the patient to ED. If the patient has attempted suicide, take them to ED.

Mental Capacity Assessment in Brief

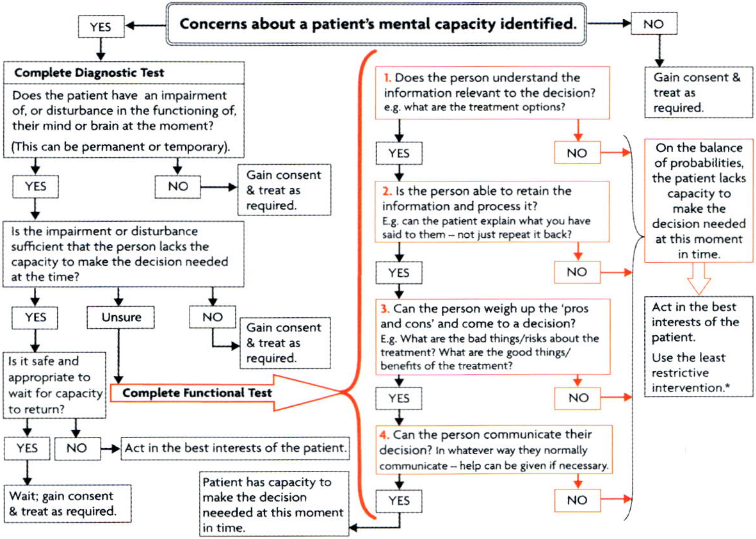

GENERAL

Concerns about a patient's mental capacity identified.

YES

NO → Gain consent & treat as required.

Complete Diagnostic Test

Does the patient have an impairment of, or disturbance in the functioning of, their mind or brain at the moment?

(This can be permanent or temporary).

YES

NO → Gain consent & treat as required.

Is the impairment or disturbance sufficient that the person lacks the capacity to make the decision needed at the time?

YES — Unsure — NO → Gain consent & treat as required.

Is it safe and appropriate to wait for capacity to return?

Complete Functional Test

YES — NO → Act in the best interests of the patient.

Wait; gain consent & treat as required.

Patient has capacity to make the decision neeeded at this moment in time.

1. Does the person understand the information relevant to the decision? e.g. what are the treatment options?

YES — NO

2. Is the person able to retain the information and process it? E.g. can the patient explain what you have said to them – not just repeat it back?

YES — NO

3. Can the person weigh up the 'pros and cons' and come to a decision? E.g. What are the bad things/risks about the treatment? What are the good things/benefits of the treatment?

YES — NO

4. Can the person communicate their decision? In whatever way they normally communicate – help can be given if necessary.

YES — NO

On the balance of probabilities, the patient lacks capacity to make the decision needed at this moment in time.

Act in the best interests of the patient.

Use the least restrictive intervention.*

* Is there a relevant substitute decision maker available? (LPA/Attorney/Court-Appointed Deputy). Is there a valid & applicable Advance Decision to refuse treatment?

Reproduced with permission of S Putman.

MEDICAL

MEDICAL

Adult Bradycardia Algorithm

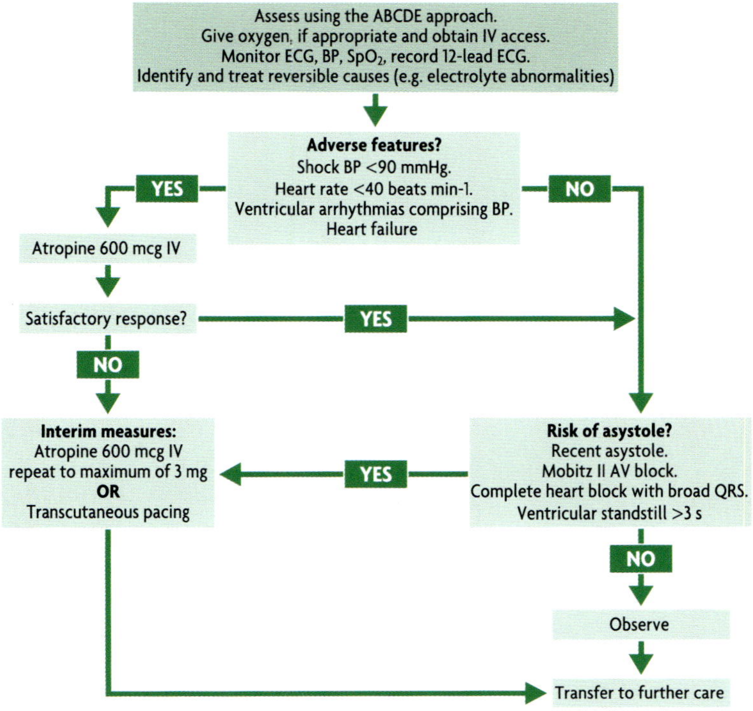

Assess using the ABCDE approach.
Give oxygen, if appropriate and obtain IV access.
Monitor ECG, BP, SpO$_2$, record 12-lead ECG.
Identify and treat reversible causes (e.g. electrolyte abnormalities)

↓

Adverse features?
Shock BP <90 mmHg.
Heart rate <40 beats min-1.
Ventricular arrhythmias comprising BP.
Heart failure

YES →

Atropine 600 mcg IV

↓

Satisfactory response? — **YES** →

NO ↓

Interim measures:
Atropine 600 mcg IV
repeat to maximum of 3 mg
OR
Transcutaneous pacing

← **YES** —

NO →

Risk of asystole?
Recent asystole.
Mobitz II AV block.
Complete heart block with broad QRS.
Ventricular standstill >3 s

NO ↓

Observe

↓

Transfer to further care

Adult Tachycardia (With Pulse)

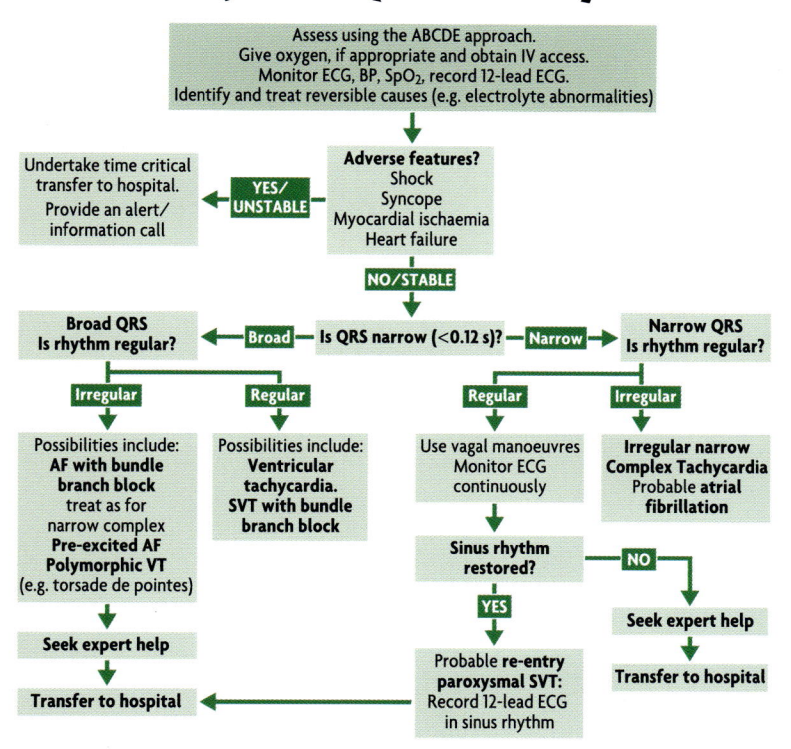

Assess using the ABCDE approach.
Give oxygen, if appropriate and obtain IV access.
Monitor ECG, BP, SpO$_2$, record 12-lead ECG.
Identify and treat reversible causes (e.g. electrolyte abnormalities)

Adverse features?
- Shock
- Syncope
- Myocardial ischaemia
- Heart failure

YES/UNSTABLE → Undertake time critical transfer to hospital. Provide an alert/information call

NO/STABLE ↓

Is QRS narrow (<0.12 s)?

Broad → **Broad QRS — Is rhythm regular?**

- **Irregular**: Possibilities include: AF with bundle branch block — treat as for narrow complex. **Pre-excited AF**, **Polymorphic VT** (e.g. torsade de pointes) → Seek expert help → Transfer to hospital
- **Regular**: Possibilities include: **Ventricular tachycardia**. **SVT with bundle branch block**

Narrow → **Narrow QRS — Is rhythm regular?**

- **Regular**: Use vagal manoeuvres. Monitor ECG continuously. **Sinus rhythm restored?**
  - **YES** → Probable re-entry paroxysmal SVT: Record 12-lead ECG in sinus rhythm
  - **NO** → Seek expert help → Transfer to hospital
- **Irregular**: **Irregular narrow Complex Tachycardia** Probable **atrial fibrillation**

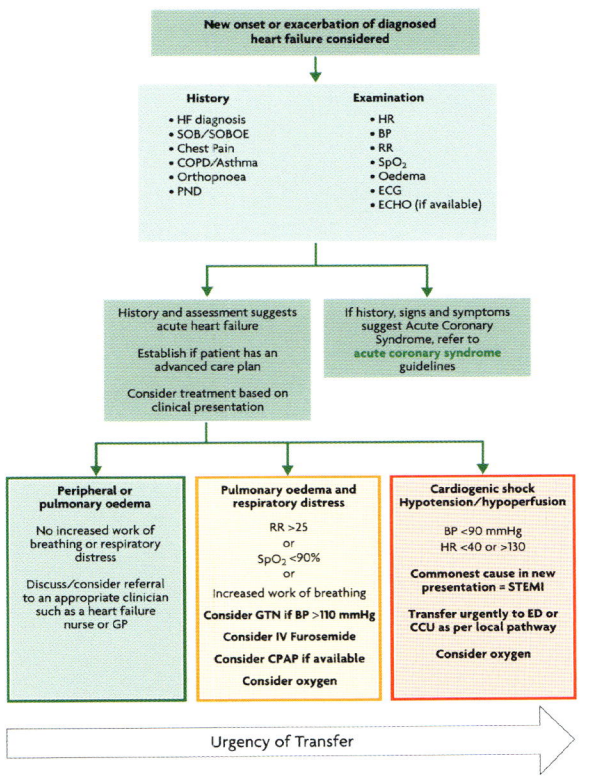

MEDICAL

Heart Failure

New onset or exacerbation of diagnosed heart failure considered

History
- HF diagnosis
- SOB/SOBOE
- Chest Pain
- COPD/Asthma
- Orthopnoea
- PND

Examination
- HR
- BP
- RR
- SpO₂
- Oedema
- ECG
- ECHO (if available)

History and assessment suggests acute heart failure

Establish if patient has an advanced care plan

Consider treatment based on clinical presentation

If history, signs and symptoms suggest Acute Coronary Syndrome, refer to acute coronary syndrome guidelines

---

Peripheral or pulmonary oedema
- No increased work of breathing or respiratory distress
- Discuss/consider referral to an appropriate clinician such as a heart failure nurse or GP

Pulmonary oedema and respiratory distress
- RR >25
or
- SpO₂ <90%
or
- Increased work of breathing
- Consider GTN if BP >110 mmHg
- Consider IV Furosemide
- Consider CPAP if available
- Consider oxygen

Cardiogenic shock Hypotension/hypoperfusion
- BP <90 mmHg
- HR <40 or <130
- Commonest cause in new presentation = STEMI
- Transfer urgently to ED or CCU as per local pathway
- Consider oxygen

← Urgency of Transfer

Pulmonary Embolism

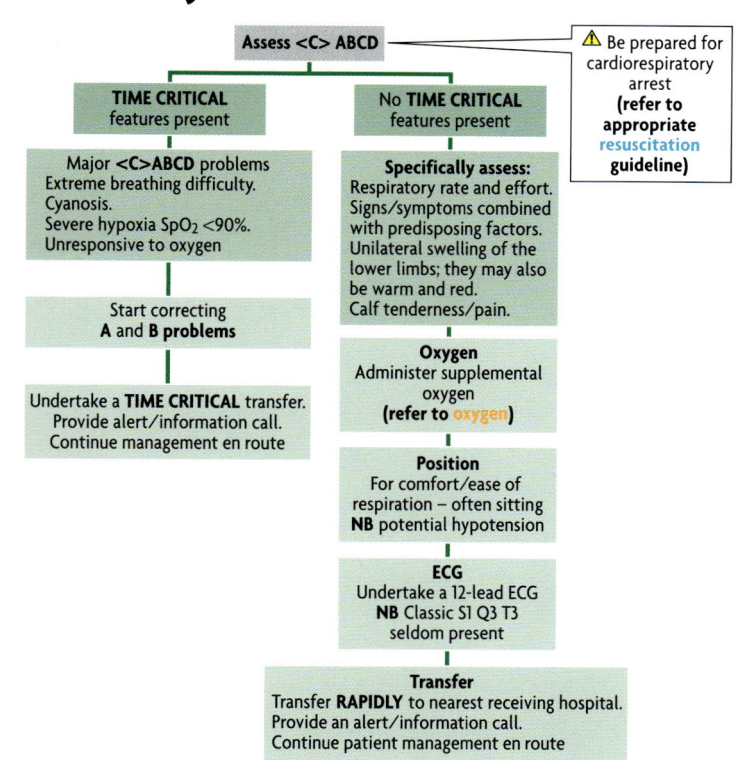

Assess <C> ABCD

⚠️ Be prepared for cardiorespiratory arrest **(refer to appropriate resuscitation guideline)**

TIME CRITICAL features present

Major **<C>ABCD** problems
Extreme breathing difficulty.
Cyanosis.
Severe hypoxia SpO$_2$ <90%.
Unresponsive to oxygen

Start correcting **A** and **B** problems

Undertake a **TIME CRITICAL** transfer.
Provide alert/information call.
Continue management en route

No TIME CRITICAL features present

Specifically assess:
Respiratory rate and effort.
Signs/symptoms combined with predisposing factors.
Unilateral swelling of the lower limbs; they may also be warm and red.
Calf tenderness/pain.

Oxygen
Administer supplemental oxygen
(refer to oxygen)

Position
For comfort/ease of respiration – often sitting
NB potential hypotension

ECG
Undertake a 12-lead ECG
NB Classic S1 Q3 T3 seldom present

Transfer
Transfer **RAPIDLY** to nearest receiving hospital.
Provide an alert/information call.
Continue patient management en route

MEDICAL

Asthma

MILD/ MODERATE ASTHMA	Move to a calm, quiet environment
	Encourage use of own inhaler, preferably using a spacer. Ensure correct technique is used; two puffs, followed by two puffs every 2 minutes to a maximum of ten puffs
	Administer high levels of supplementary **oxygen**
	Administer nebulised **salbutamol** using an oxygen driven nebuliser **(refer to salbutamol)**
SEVERE ASTHMA	If no improvement, administer **ipratropium bromide** by nebuliser **(refer to ipratropium bromide)**
	Administer steroids **(refer to relevant steroids guideline)**
	Continuous **salbutamol** nebulisation may be administered unless clinically significant side effects occur **(refer to salbutamol)**
LIFE-THREATENING ASTHMA	Administer **adrenaline** **(refer to adrenaline)**
	Assess for bilateral tension pneumothorax and treat if present. Provide an alert/information call
NEAR-FATAL ASTHMA	As you progress through the treatment algorithm consider the patient's overall response on the condition arrow and transfer as indicated

IMPROVING

CONSIDER TRANSFER

DETERIORATING

TIME CRITICAL TRANSFER

Asthma Features of Severity

Near-fatal asthma
- Raised $PaCO_2$ and/or requiring mechanical ventilation with raised inflation pressures.

Life-threatening asthma
Any one of the following in a patient with severe asthma:
- Altered conscious level.
- Exhaustion.
- Arrhythmia.
- Hypotension.
- Cyanosis.
- Silent chest.
- Poor respiratory effort.
- PEF <33% best or predicted.
- SpO_2 <92%.
- PaO_2 <8 kPa.
- 'Abnormal' $PaCO_2$ (Normal range: 4.6–6.0 kPa).

Acute severe asthma
Any one of:
- PEF 33–50% best or predicted.
- Inability to complete sentences in one breath.
- Pulse:
  - >110/minute in adults
  - >125/minute in children >5 years
  - >140/minute in children 2-5 years
- Respiration:
  - >25/minute in adults
  - >30/minute in children >5 years
  - >40/minute in children 2-5 years

Mild/moderate asthma exacerbation
- Able to speak in sentences.
- Increasing symptoms.
- PEF >50–75% best or predicted.
- No features of acute severe asthma.
- Heart rate:
  - ≤140/min in children aged 2–5 years.
  - ≤125/min in children >5 years.
- Respiratory rate:
  - ≤40/min in children aged 2–5 years.
  - ≤30/min in children >5 years.

MEDICAL

Asthma Peak Flow Charts

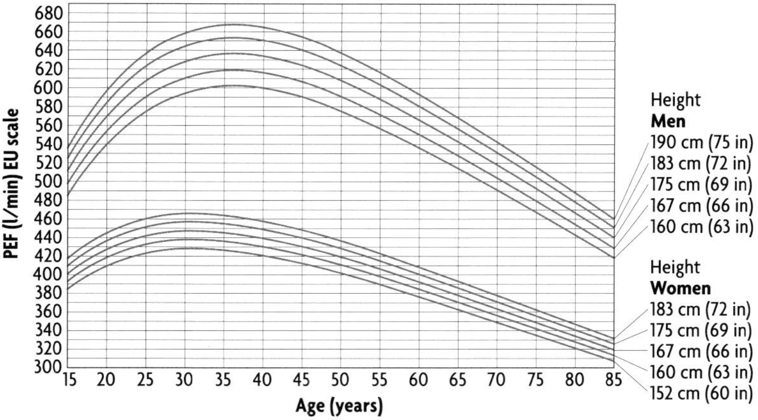

Peak flow charts – Peak expiratory flow rate – normal values. For use with EU/EN13826 scale PEF meters only.*

* Adapted by Clement Clarke for use with EN13826 / EU scale peak flow meters from Nunn AJ, Gregg I: Br Med J 1989:298;1068-70.

Chronic Obstructive Pulmonary Disease

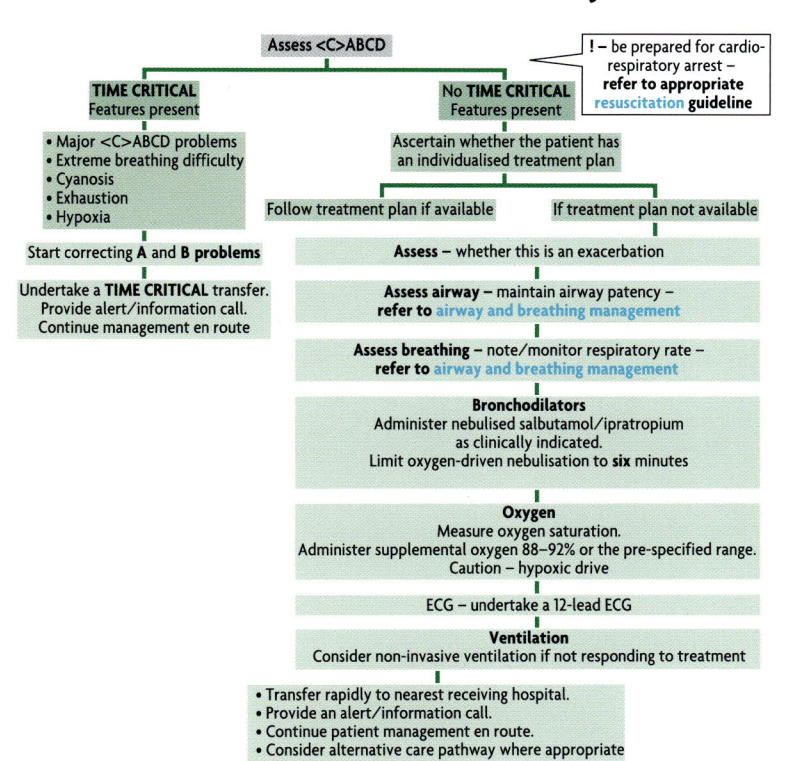

Assess <C>ABCD

> ! – be prepared for cardio-respiratory arrest – **refer to appropriate resuscitation guideline**

TIME CRITICAL Features present

- Major <C>ABCD problems
- Extreme breathing difficulty
- Cyanosis
- Exhaustion
- Hypoxia

Start correcting **A** and **B** problems

Undertake a TIME CRITICAL transfer.
Provide alert/information call.
Continue management en route

No TIME CRITICAL Features present

Ascertain whether the patient has an individualised treatment plan

- Follow treatment plan if available
- If treatment plan not available

Assess – whether this is an exacerbation

Assess airway – maintain airway patency – **refer to** airway and breathing management

Assess breathing – note/monitor respiratory rate – **refer to** airway and breathing management

Bronchodilators
Administer nebulised salbutamol/ipratropium as clinically indicated.
Limit oxygen-driven nebulisation to **six** minutes

Oxygen
Measure oxygen saturation.
Administer supplemental oxygen 88–92% or the pre-specified range.
Caution – hypoxic drive

ECG – undertake a 12-lead ECG

Ventilation
Consider non-invasive ventilation if not responding to treatment

- Transfer rapidly to nearest receiving hospital.
- Provide an alert/information call.
- Continue patient management en route.
- Consider alternative care pathway where appropriate

Convulsions (Adults)

MEDICAL

CONVULSION(S) ONGOING OR RECURRENT

Continue to assess <C>ABCDE
Consider/treat cause:
hypoxia, hypoglycaemia (check blood glucose), epilepsy, PNES, eclampsia or convulsion provoked by: head injury, stroke, alcohol, drug overdose or infection

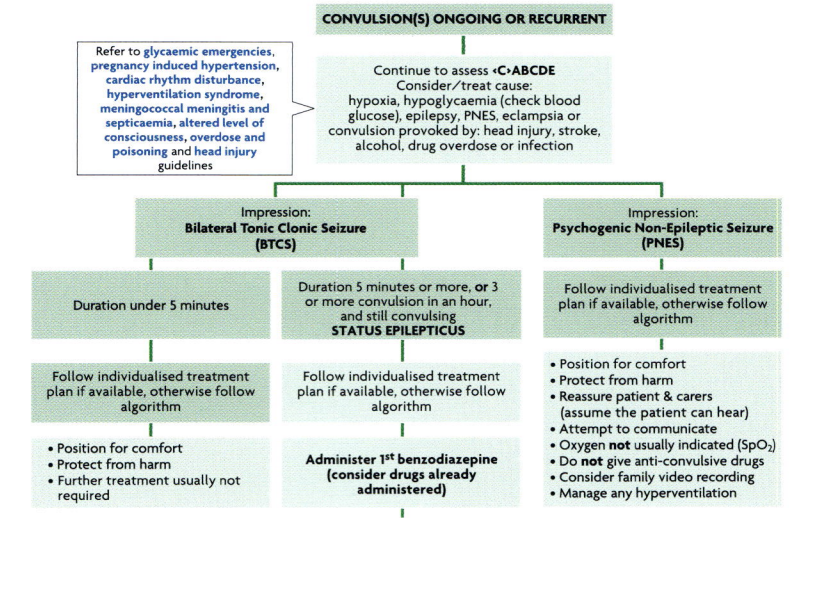

Refer to glycaemic emergencies, pregnancy induced hypertension, cardiac rhythm disturbance, meningococcal meningitis and hyperventilation syndrome, septicaemia, altered level of consciousness, overdose and poisoning and head injury guidelines

---

Impression: Bilateral Tonic Clonic Seizure (BTCS)

Duration under 5 minutes

- Position for comfort
- Protect from harm
- Further treatment usually not required

Follow individualised treatment plan if available, otherwise follow algorithm

---

Duration 5 minutes or more, or 3 or more convulsion in an hour, and still convulsing

STATUS EPILEPTICUS

Administer 1st benzodiazepine (consider drugs already administered)

Follow individualised treatment plan if available, otherwise follow algorithm

---

Impression: Psychogenic Non-Epileptic Seizure (PNES)

- Position for comfort
- Protect from harm
- Reassure patient & carers
- Attempt to communicate (assume the patient can hear)
- Oxygen **not** usually indicated (SpO$_2$)
- **Do not** give anti-convulsive drugs
- Consider family video recording
- Manage any hyperventilation

Follow individualised treatment plan if available, otherwise follow algorithm

Convulsions (Adults)

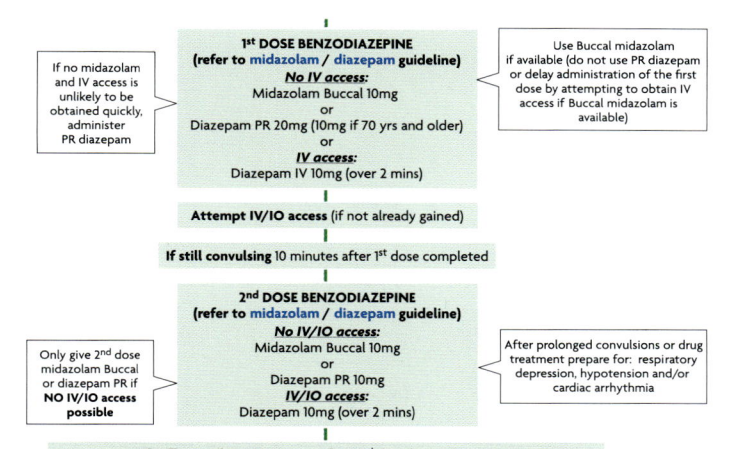

1st DOSE BENZODIAZEPINE
(refer to midazolam / diazepam guideline)
No IV access:
Midazolam Buccal 10mg
or
Diazepam PR 20mg (10mg if 70 yrs and older)
or
IV access:
Diazepam IV 10mg (over 2 mins)

If no midazolam and IV access is unlikely to be obtained quickly, administer PR diazepam

Use Buccal midazolam if available (do not use PR diazepam or delay administration of the first dose by attempting to obtain IV access if Buccal midazolam is available)

Attempt IV/IO access (if not already gained)

If still convulsing 10 minutes after 1st dose completed

2nd DOSE BENZODIAZEPINE
(refer to midazolam / diazepam guideline)
No IV/IO access:
Midazolam Buccal 10mg
or
Diazepam PR 10mg
or
IV/IO access:
Diazepam 10mg (over 2 mins)

*Only give 2nd dose midazolam Buccal or diazepam PR if **NO IV/IO access possible***

After prolonged convulsions or drug treatment prepare for: respiratory depression, hypotension and/or cardiac arrhythmia

If still convulsing 10 minutes after 2nd dose benzodiazepine:
Seek senior clinical advice to consider diagnosis (is this a PNES?), and risk/benefit of 3rd dose IV/IO benzodiazepine (en-route) if **no** alternative anticonvulsant available **and** still another 15 minutes or more from hospital (i.e. total 25 minutes from end of last dose)

47

MEDICAL

Glycaemic Emergencies (Adults)

MILD	MODERATE	SEVERE
The patient is conscious, orientated and able to swallow.	The patient is conscious and able to swallow, but may be confused, disoriented and/or combative.	The patient is unconscious/fitting or combative or where there is increased risk of aspiration/choking.

MILD

- Give 15–20 g quick acting carbohydrate, such as:
    - 4–5 Glucotabs or
    - 1 bottle (60 ml) Glucojuice® or
    - 1–2 tubes 40% glucose gel or
    - 3–4 heaped teaspoons of sugar dissolved in water or
    - 150–200 ml pure fruit juice.

- Re-test blood glucose after 15 mins.

- If blood glucose remains <4 mmol/l, repeat above treatment up to twice more at 15-minute intervals until a blood glucose of >4 mmol/l is obtained.

- If blood glucose fails to rise >4 mmol/l AFTER 3 cycles of oral treatment (i.e. 45 mins), consider IV 10% glucose or IM glucagon.

MODERATE

If capable and cooperative:

- Give 15–20 g quick acting carbohydrate, such as:
    - 4–5 Glucotabs or
    - 1 bottle (60 ml) Glucojuice® or
    - 1–2 tubes 40% glucose gel or
    - 3–4 heaped teaspoons of sugar dissolved in water or
    - 150–200 ml pure fruit juice.

If **NOT** capable and cooperative, but able to swallow:

- Administer 1–2 tubes of glucose gel 40% to the buccal mucosa or give 1 mg glucagon IM (refer to Glucagon).

- Re-test blood glucose after 15 mins. If <4 mmol/l, repeat administration of 40% glucose gel. **NB** IM glucagon cannot be repeated.

SEVERE

- Check ABC and correct as necessary.

- Administer IV glucose 10% over 15 minutes (refer to Glucose 10% for dosages).

- If IV not possible administer IM glucagon (may take up to 15 minutes to work and IM glucagon ONCE ONLY).

- Re-assess blood glucose level after 10 minutes.

- If blood glucose remains <4.0 mmol/l, administer a further dose of IV 10% glucose.

- Repeat treatment until a blood glucose of >4 mmol/l is obtained.

Glycaemic Emergencies (Adults)

- If 40% glucose gel cannot be administered due to patient disposition, consider IV 10% glucose (refer to Glucose 10%).
- If blood glucose remains <4 mmol/l, repeat above treatment up to twice more at 15-minute intervals until a blood glucose of >4 mmol/l is obtained.

- If no improvement, convey to nearest suitable receiving hospital.
- Check glucose again if patient deteriorates.
- Provide a pre-alert/information call if necessary.

Blood glucose level should now be 4 mmol/l or above.

- Once a blood glucose of >4 mmol/l is achieved, give a starchy snack, e.g. two biscuits; one slice of bread/toast; 200–300 ml glass of milk (not soya); a normal meal if due (must contain carbohydrate).
- **NB** Patients given glucagon require a larger portion of long-acting carbohydrate to replenish glycogen stores (double the suggested amount above).
- **NB** Patients who self-manage their insulin pumps (CSII) may not need a long-acting carbohydrate.
- In most cases patients who have fully recovered and maintain glucose levels >4 mmol/l will not require admission to ED.

If blood glucose is now >4 mmol/l, follow up treatment as described on the left.

Glucagon may take up to 15 minutes to work and can be ineffective in the very young, older people, undernourished patients or those with hepatic disease.
In patients with renal/cardiac disease, use IV fluids with caution.
Avoid fruit juice in renal failure. **Note:** the carbohydrate content of some commercially available glucose-containing drinks varies – individual product labels should be checked. Diet drinks may not contain sugar.

MEDICAL

Allergic Reactions including Anaphylaxis

Quickly remove from trigger if possible (e.g. environmental, infusion etc.)
DO NOT delay definitive treatment if removing trigger not feasible

Assess <C>ABCDE
If **TIME CRITICAL** features present – correct **A** and **B** and transfer to nearest appropriate receiving hospital. **Provide an ATMIST information call**

Consider mild/moderate allergic reaction if:
onset of illness is minutes to hours
AND
cutaneous findings (e.g. urticaria and/or angio-oedema)

Consider chlorphenamine
(refer to chlorphenamine)

Consider anaphylaxis if:
Sudden onset and rapid progression
Airway and/or **Breathing problems** (e.g. dyspnoea, hoarseness, stridor, wheeze, throat or chest tightness) and/or **Circulation** (e.g. hypotension, syncope, pronounced tachycardia) and/or **Skin** (e.g. erythema, urticaria, mucosal changes) problems

Administer high levels of supplementary oxygen and aim for a target saturation of >94% **(refer to oxygen)**

⚠ **Intramuscular** adrenaline only

Administer 1:1,000 **IM** adrenaline **(refer to adrenaline)**

If haemodynamically compromised consider fluid therapy **(refer to fluid therapy)**

Consider chlorphenamine **(refer to chlorphenamine)**

Consider administering hydrocortisone **(refer to hydrocortisone)**

Consider nebulised salbutamol for bronchospasm **(refer to salbutamol)**

Monitor and re-assess ABC
Monitor ECG, PEFR (if possible), BP and pulse oximetry en-route

Sickle Cell Crisis

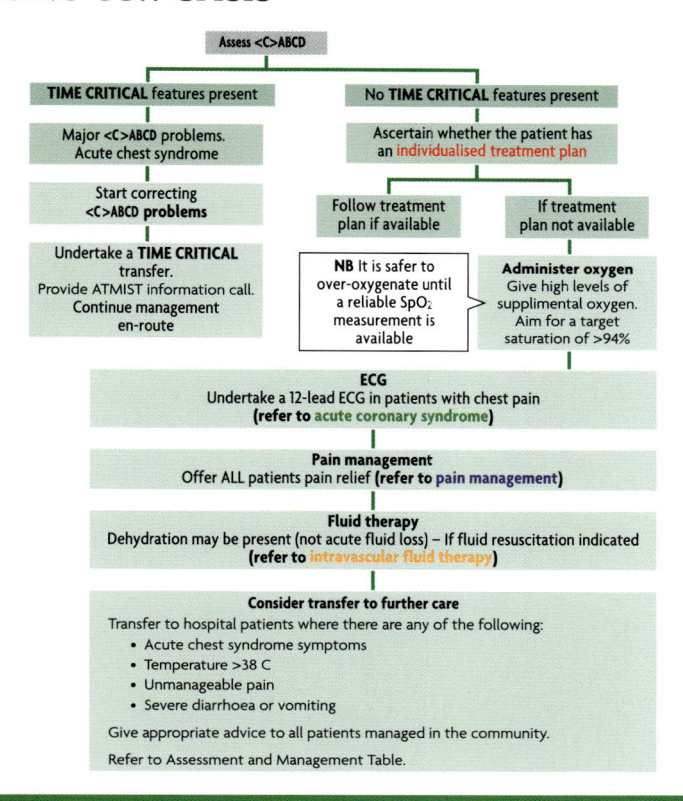

Assess <C>ABCD

TIME CRITICAL features present

Major <C>ABCD problems.
Acute chest syndrome

Start correcting <C>ABCD problems

Undertake a **TIME CRITICAL** transfer.
Provide ATMIST information call.
Continue management en-route

No TIME CRITICAL features present

Ascertain whether the patient has an individualised treatment plan

- Follow treatment plan if available
- If treatment plan not available

NB It is safer to over-oxygenate until a reliable SpO_2 measurement is available

Administer oxygen
Give high levels of supplemental oxygen. Aim for a target saturation of >94%

ECG
Undertake a 12-lead ECG in patients with chest pain
(refer to acute coronary syndrome)

Pain management
Offer ALL patients pain relief **(refer to pain management)**

Fluid therapy
Dehydration may be present (not acute fluid loss) – If fluid resuscitation indicated
(refer to intravascular fluid therapy)

Consider transfer to further care
Transfer to hospital patients where there are any of the following:
- Acute chest syndrome symptoms
- Temperature >38 C
- Unmanageable pain
- Severe diarrhoea or vomiting

Give appropriate advice to all patients managed in the community.

Refer to Assessment and Management Table.

TRAUMA

Trauma – ATMIST

ATMIST	
A	Age
T	Time of incident
M	Mechanism
I	Injuries
S	Signs and symptoms
T	Treatment given/immediate needs

Trauma Survey

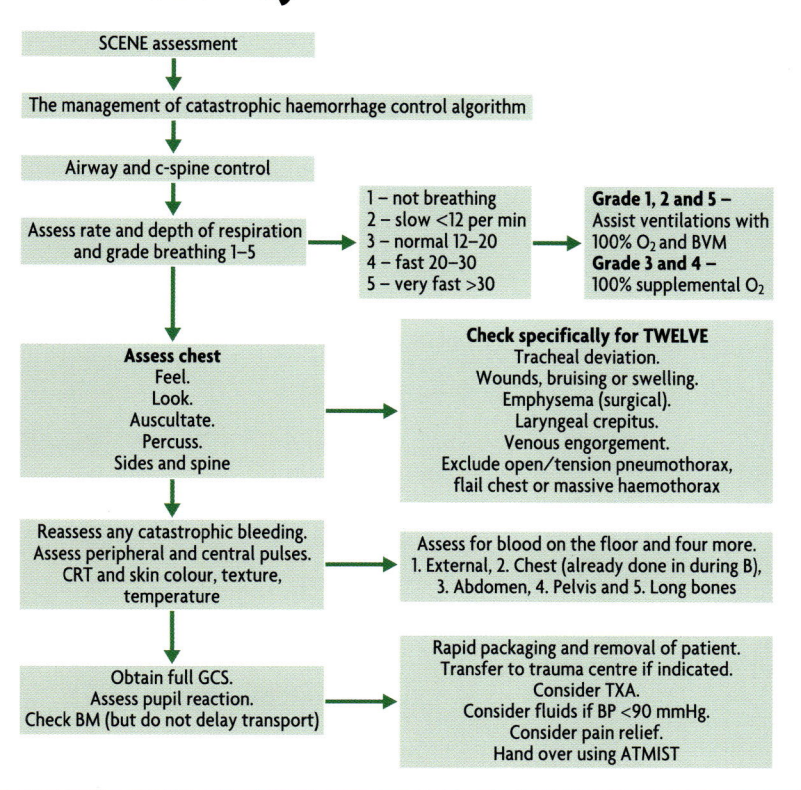

```
SCENE assessment
        ↓
The management of catastrophic haemorrhage control algorithm
        ↓
Airway and c-spine control
        ↓
Assess rate and depth of respiration
and grade breathing 1–5
```

- 1 – not breathing
- 2 – slow <12 per min
- 3 – normal 12–20
- 4 – fast 20–30
- 5 – very fast >30

Grade 1, 2 and 5 – Assist ventilations with 100% O_2 and BVM
Grade 3 and 4 – 100% supplemental O_2

Assess chest
Feel.
Look.
Auscultate.
Percuss.
Sides and spine.

Check specifically for TWELVE
Tracheal deviation.
Wounds, bruising or swelling.
Emphysema (surgical).
Laryngeal crepitus.
Venous engorgement.
Exclude open/tension pneumothorax, flail chest or massive haemothorax

Reassess any catastrophic bleeding.
Assess peripheral and central pulses.
CRT and skin colour, texture, temperature

Assess for blood on the floor and four more.
1. External, 2. Chest (already done in during B), 3. Abdomen, 4. Pelvis and 5. Long bones

Obtain full GCS.
Assess pupil reaction.
Check BM (but do not delay transport)

Rapid packaging and removal of patient.
Transfer to trauma centre if indicated.
Consider TXA.
Consider fluids if BP <90 mmHg.
Consider pain relief.
Hand over using ATMIST

55

TRAUMA

Trauma Emergencies Overview (Adults)

The management of haemorrhage algorithm.

Haemorrhage

Apply a field dressing

Apply direct pressure

NB Pressure must be firm and applied directly over the wound

Where possible elevate the bleeding point above heart height

Bleeding controlled

Transfer to further care

Bleeding NOT controlled

Apply further dressings and continue to apply direct pressure

Bleeding controlled

Transfer to further care

Bleeding NOT controlled

Refer to catastrophic haemorrhage management – **start at appropriate point**

A

Jump to **point A** on the head, neck, torso side of the catastrophic haemorrhage algorithm

B

Jump to **point B** on the limbs side of the catastrophic haemorrhage algorithm

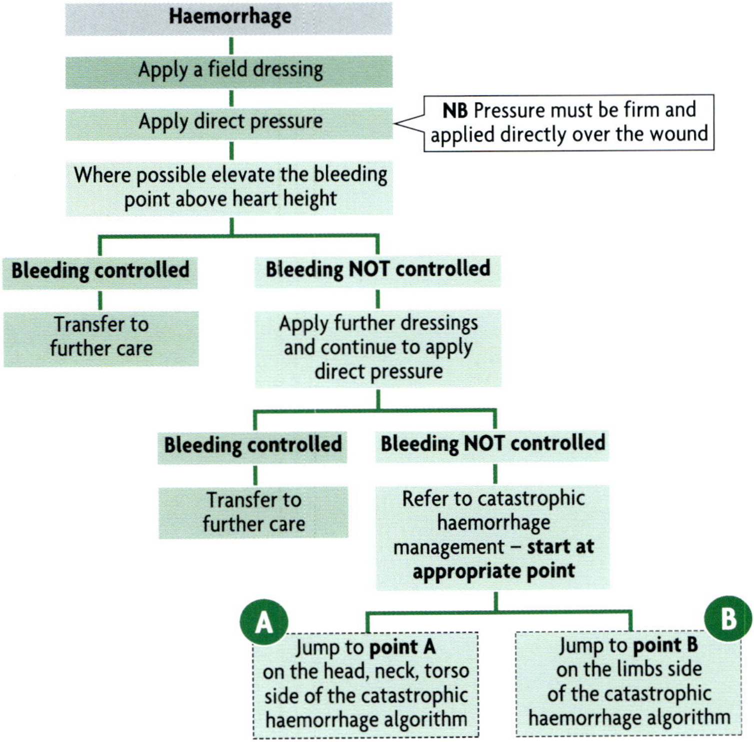

Trauma Emergencies Overview (Adults)

The management of catastrophic haemorrhage algorithm.

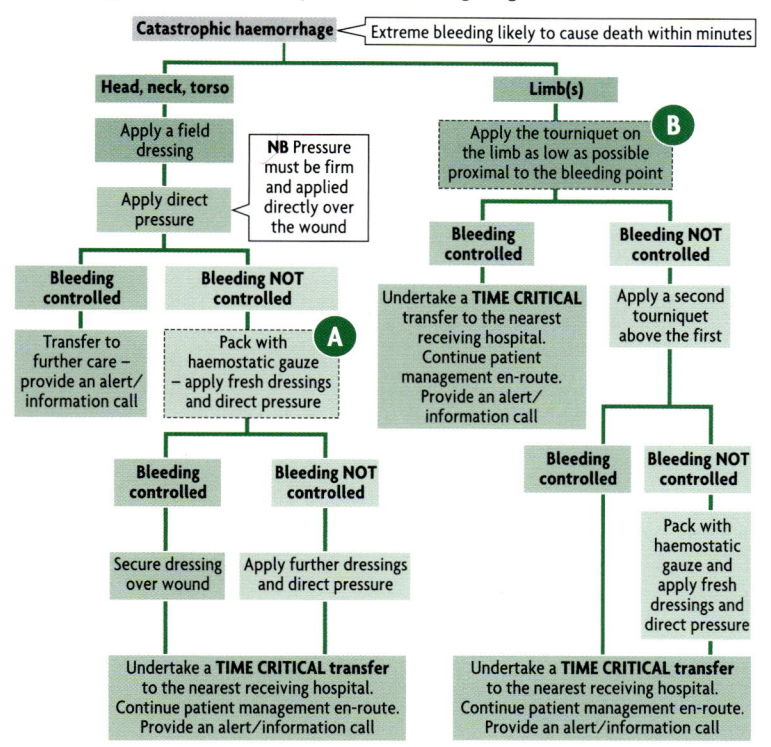

Catastrophic haemorrhage — Extreme bleeding likely to cause death within minutes

Head, neck, torso

- Apply a field dressing
- Apply direct pressure

NB Pressure must be firm and applied directly over the wound

Bleeding controlled
Transfer to further care – provide an alert/information call

Bleeding NOT controlled
Pack with haemostatic gauze – apply fresh dressings and direct pressure **A**

Bleeding controlled
Secure dressing over wound

Bleeding NOT controlled
Apply further dressings and direct pressure

Undertake a **TIME CRITICAL** transfer to the nearest receiving hospital. Continue patient management en-route. Provide an alert/information call

Limb(s)

Apply the tourniquet on the limb as low as possible proximal to the bleeding point **B**

Bleeding controlled
Undertake a **TIME CRITICAL** transfer to the nearest receiving hospital. Continue patient management en-route. Provide an alert/information call

Bleeding NOT controlled
Apply a second tourniquet above the first

Bleeding controlled

Bleeding NOT controlled
Pack with haemostatic gauze and apply fresh dressings and direct pressure

Undertake a **TIME CRITICAL** transfer to the nearest receiving hospital. Continue patient management en-route. Provide an alert/information call

TRAUMA

Spinal Injury and Spinal Cord Injury

Patients with a history of trauma
Is there a potential for spinal injury in an adult >16 years old?

Yes

- Under the influence of drugs or alcohol?
- Is confused or uncooperative?
- Has a reduced level of consciousness?
- Has any spinal pain (or pain elicited on coughing)?
- Any motor weakness in hands or feet?
- Any history of past spinal problems, including previous spinal surgery, severe osteoarthritis, ankylosing spondylitis?
- Any priapism?

No

High Risk?
- Dangerous mechanism of injury (fall from a height of >1 metre or five steps, axial load to the head - e.g. diving, high-speed motor vehicle collision, rollover motor accident, ejection from a motor vehicle, accident involving motorised recreational vehicles, bicycle collision, horse riding accidents)

No

Use of spinal immobilisation devices may be difficult (e.g. in people with short/wide necks, or people with a pre-existing deformity) and could be counterproductive (i.e. increasing pain, worsening neurological signs and symptoms). In uncooperative, agitated or distressed people, think about letting them find a position where they are comfortable with manual in-line spinal immobilisation

Yes

*Immobilise the entire spine. If the patient is ambulatory or has been ambulatory at the scene, they can self-extricate if appropriate and may be guided to lie down onto the scoop stretcher to be immobilised. The scoop should be placed on the trolley and located as close as practicable to the patient. Patients MUST NOT be encouraged to walk up any steps (causes potential axial loading).

Yes

IMMOBILISE*

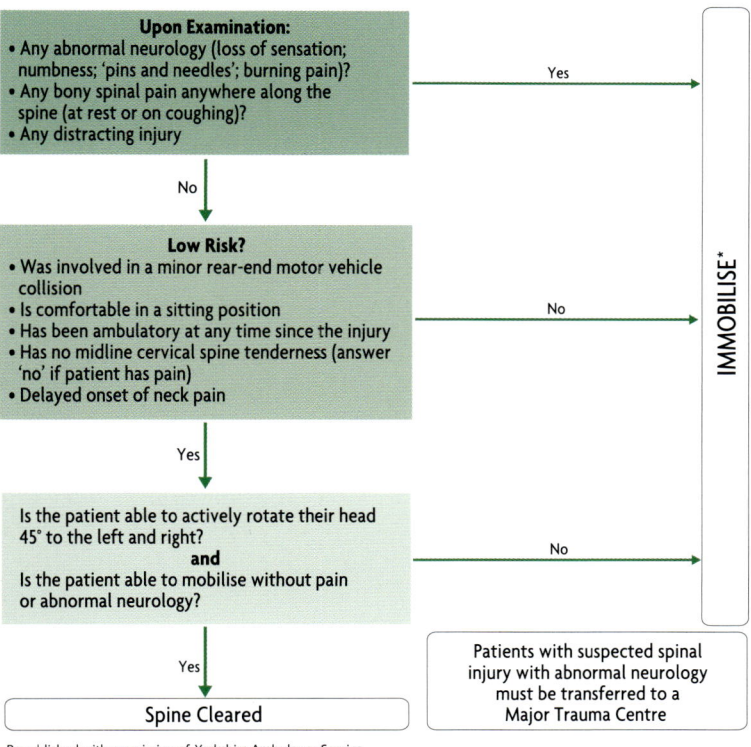

```
                    ┌─────────────────────────────────────────────┐
                    │ Upon Examination:                           │
                    │ • Any abnormal neurology (loss of sensation;│────── Yes ──────┐
                    │   numbness; 'pins and needles'; burning pain)?│              │
                    │ • Any bony spinal pain anywhere along the   │                │
                    │   spine (at rest or on coughing)?           │                │
                    │ • Any distracting injury                    │                │
                    └─────────────────────────────────────────────┘                │
                                         │ No                                      │
                    ┌─────────────────────────────────────────────┐                │
                    │ Low Risk?                                   │                │
                    │ • Was involved in a minor rear-end motor    │                │
                    │   vehicle collision                         │                │
                    │ • Is comfortable in a sitting position      │────── No ──────┤
                    │ • Has been ambulatory at any time since     │                │
                    │   the injury                                │             IMMOBILISE*
                    │ • Has no midline cervical spine tenderness  │                │
                    │   (answer 'no' if patient has pain)         │                │
                    │ • Delayed onset of neck pain                │                │
                    └─────────────────────────────────────────────┘                │
                                         │ Yes                                     │
                    ┌─────────────────────────────────────────────┐                │
                    │ Is the patient able to actively rotate their│                │
                    │ head 45° to the left and right?             │                │
                    │                  and                        │────── No ──────┘
                    │ Is the patient able to mobilise without pain│
                    │ or abnormal neurology?                      │
                    └─────────────────────────────────────────────┘
                                         │ Yes
                              ┌──────────────────────┐
                              │    Spine Cleared     │
                              └──────────────────────┘
```

Patients with suspected spinal injury with abnormal neurology must be transferred to a Major Trauma Centre

Republished with permission of Yorkshire Ambulance Service

SPECIAL SITUATIONS

SP SITU

METHANE Report Format

METHANE Report Format

M   Major incident standby or declared

E   Exact location of incident

T   Type of incident

H   Hazards (present and potential)

A   Access and egress routes

N   Number, severity and type of casualties

E   Emergency services present on scene and further resources required

For a major incident, now follow your Major Incident Action Cards

Triage Sieve

Triage Sieve

Best practice is to carry out TRIAGE SIEVE in pairs

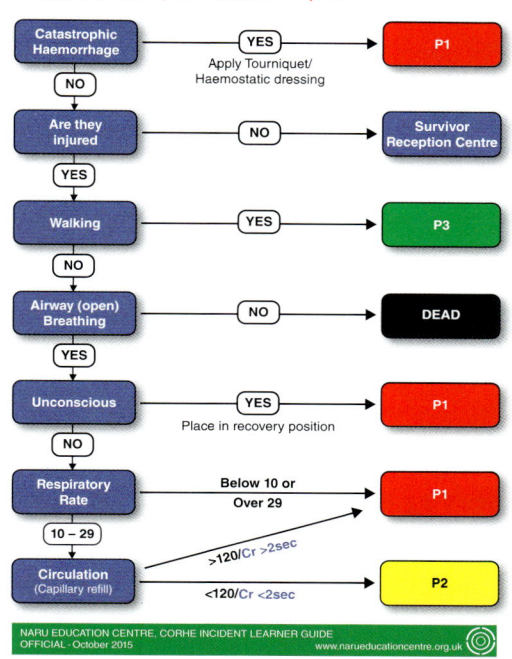

- **Catastrophic Haemorrhage** — YES → Apply Tourniquet/Haemostatic dressing → **P1**
- NO ↓
- **Are they injured** — NO → **Survivor Reception Centre**
- YES ↓
- **Walking** — YES → **P3**
- NO ↓
- **Airway (open) Breathing** — NO → **DEAD**
- YES ↓
- **Unconscious** — YES → Place in recovery position → **P1**
- NO ↓
- **Respiratory Rate** — Below 10 or Over 29 → **P1**
- 10 – 29 ↓
- **Circulation (Capillary refill)** — >120/Cr >2sec → **P1**; <120/Cr <2sec → **P2**

NARU EDUCATION CENTRE, CORHE INCIDENT LEARNER GUIDE
OFFICIAL - October 2015   www.narueducationcentre.org.uk

SP SITU

Specialist Capabilities

When responding to a complex or high-risk incident, it is essential for ambulance staff to request these specialist services early. They can be easily stood down if not required.

The tactical options of different core capabilities are listed below.

HART: Hazardous Area Response Teams

Hazardous Materials: Working inside the inner cordon, industrial accidents, high-risk infectious diseases and complex transportation accidents.

Chemical, Biological, Radiological, Nuclear and Explosives – CBRN(e): Specialist operational response (SOR), also a component part of the wider CBRN(e) capability.

Marauding Terrorist Attack – MTA: Specialist support to warm zone operations/component part of wider MTA capability.

Safe Working at Height – (SWaH): Manmade structures and natural environment.

Confined Space: Substantially enclosed spaces, building collapses, compromised atmospheres and entrapments.

Unstable Terrain: Active rubble piles and rural access/difficult terrain.

Water Operations: Swift water rescue, urban and rural flooding and boat operations.

Support to Security Operations: Support to security operations, support to Police operations, illicit drug laboratories and VIP close protection support.

MTFA: Marauding Terrorist Attack
- Working inside a ballistically unsafe area (warm zone)
- Siege/stronghold

CBRN(e): Chemical, Biological, Radiological, Nuclear and Explosives
- Initial Operational Response (IOR)
- Specialist Operational Response (SOR - provided by HART)
- Interim decontamination of casualties
- Full wet decontamination of casualties

C2: Command and Control
- Strategic command of major and critical incidents
- Tactical command of major and critical incidents
- Operational command of major and critical incidents
- National Interagency Liaison Officers (NILOs)
- Strategic and tactical advisors
- Medical advisors

Mass Casualties
- Capabilities to treat large numbers of casualties
- Casualty clearing stations (CCS)
- National coordination of patient transfers

MATERNITY

Maternity Care

APGAR SCORE

Score	0	1	2
Appearance	blue or pale all over	blue at extremities body pink	body and extremities pink
Pulse rate	absent	<100	≥100
Grimace or response to stimulation	no response to stimulation	grimace/ feeble cry when stimulated	cry or pull away when stimulated
Activity or muscle tone	none	some flexion	flexed arms and legs that resist extension
Respiration	absent	weak, irregular, gasping	strong, lusty cry

Breech Birth

Breech position noted in maternal notes or thick meconium seen at vaginal opening

BREECH BIRTH IMMINENT

Request midwife if available
Prepare for newborn life support

Position on edge of bed/trolley or on all fours

HANDS OFF
Allow breech to descend spontaneously with maternal pushing
DO NOT touch baby or handle umbilical cord

In either position, ensure the baby's back is always facing towards the maternal abdomen

Support baby as head births

Treat as normal birth or **refer to Newborn Life Support**

BREECH BIRTH NOT IMMINENT OR ANY OTHER PRESENTING PART (i.e. hand/arm)

Transfer to nearest appropriate destination as agreed locally
Maternal safety is the prime consideration
Consider the specific clinical situation **and which interventions may be required for the woman and baby on arrival**
Refer to 'Appropriate Destination for Conveyance' in **Maternity Care**
Continuously assess for birth imminent en-route

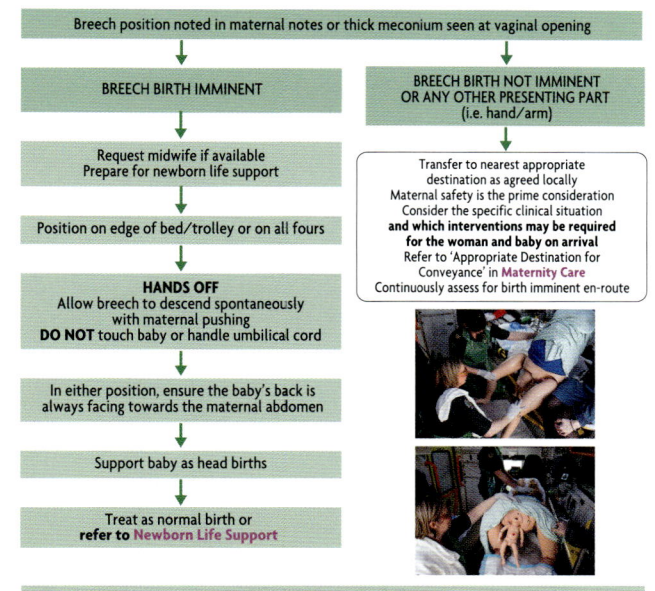

IF DELAY OCCURS DURING THE BIRTH:

LEGS: apply gentle pressure behind the baby's knee
ARMS: gently rotate the baby's pelvis 90 degrees to aid birth of the first arm – rotate the baby's body in the opposite direction if required to birth the second arm – allow the baby's body to hang unassisted
HEAD: support the baby with one arm and use the other hand to aid flexion of the back of the baby's head while delivering baby

DO NOT PULL ON THE BABY
DO NOT CLAMP AND CUT THE UMBILICAL CORD DURING THE BIRTH

MATERNITY

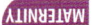

Cord Prolapse

Gently replace the umbilical cord within the opening of the vagina using a dry pad

↓

Position the woman in the knee chest position while awaiting the ambulance

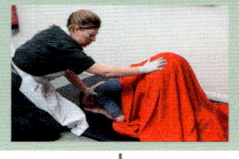

↓

Walk the woman to the ambulance

↓

Position the woman in the lateral position
Elevate the pelvis using a blanket below the right hip

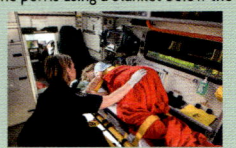

↓

Assess for imminent birth en-route
Administer Entonox if required

Transfer to nearest appropriate destination as agreed locally
Maternal safety is the prime consideration
Consider the specific clinical situation **and which interventions may be required for the woman and baby on arrival**
Refer to 'Appropriate Destination for Conveyance' in **Maternity Care**
Pre-alert stating obstetric emergency of cord prolapse
Take maternity notes if available

Eclampsia

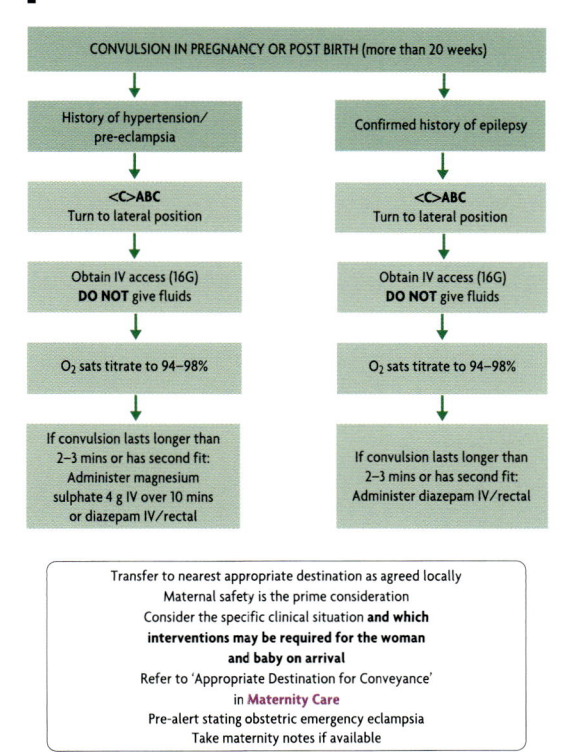

CONVULSION IN PREGNANCY OR POST BIRTH (more than 20 weeks)

History of hypertension/pre-eclampsia

↓

<C>ABC
Turn to lateral position

↓

Obtain IV access (16G)
DO NOT give fluids

↓

O_2 sats titrate to 94–98%

↓

If convulsion lasts longer than 2–3 mins or has second fit:
Administer magnesium sulphate 4 g IV over 10 mins or diazepam IV/rectal

---

Confirmed history of epilepsy

↓

<C>ABC
Turn to lateral position

↓

Obtain IV access (16G)
DO NOT give fluids

↓

O_2 sats titrate to 94–98%

↓

If convulsion lasts longer than 2–3 mins or has second fit:
Administer diazepam IV/rectal

Transfer to nearest appropriate destination as agreed locally
Maternal safety is the prime consideration
Consider the specific clinical situation **and which interventions may be required for the woman and baby on arrival**
Refer to 'Appropriate Destination for Conveyance' in **Maternity Care**
Pre-alert stating obstetric emergency eclampsia
Take maternity notes if available

MATERNITY

Newborn Life Support

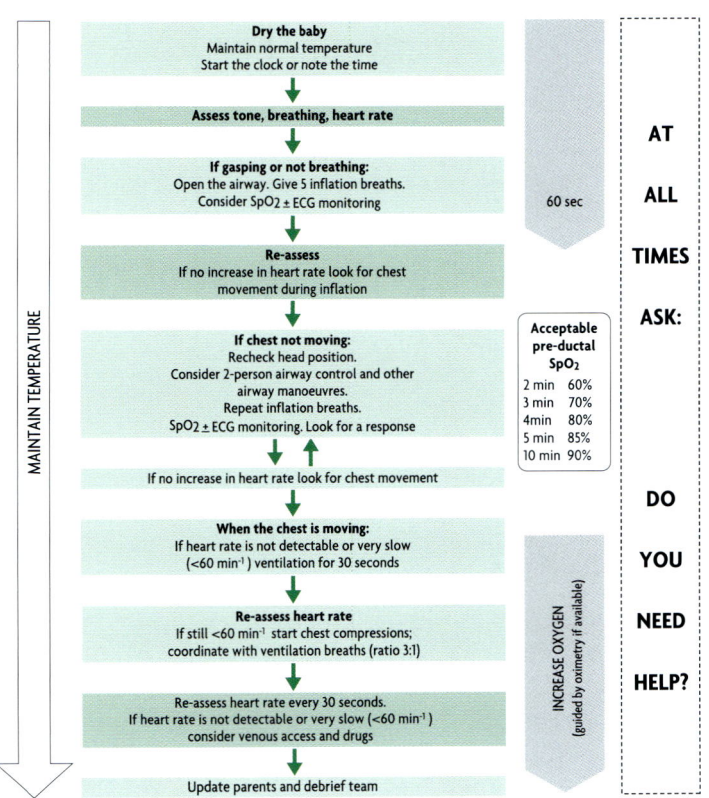

Dry the baby
Maintain normal temperature
Start the clock or note the time

↓

Assess tone, breathing, heart rate

↓

If gasping or not breathing:
Open the airway. Give 5 inflation breaths.
Consider SpO2 ± ECG monitoring

60 sec

↓

Re-assess
If no increase in heart rate look for chest movement during inflation

↓

If chest not moving:
Recheck head position.
Consider 2-person airway control and other airway manoeuvres.
Repeat inflation breaths.
SpO2 ± ECG monitoring. Look for a response

Acceptable pre-ductal SpO2
2 min	60%
3 min	70%
4 min	80%
5 min	85%
10 min	90%

↓

If no increase in heart rate look for chest movement

↓

When the chest is moving:
If heart rate is not detectable or very slow (<60 min⁻¹) ventilation for 30 seconds

↓

Re-assess heart rate
If still <60 min⁻¹ start chest compressions;
coordinate with ventilation breaths (ratio 3:1)

↓

Re-assess heart rate every 30 seconds.
If heart rate is not detectable or very slow (<60 min⁻¹)
consider venous access and drugs

↓

Update parents and debrief team

AT ALL TIMES ASK: DO YOU NEED HELP?

INCREASE OXYGEN (guided by oximetry if available)

MAINTAIN TEMPERATURE

Normal Birth

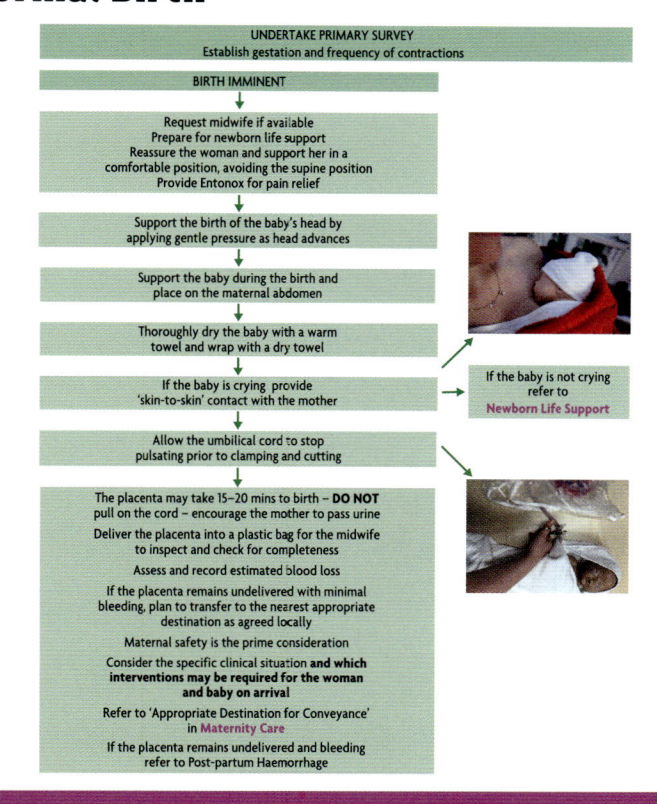

UNDERTAKE PRIMARY SURVEY
Establish gestation and frequency of contractions

↓

BIRTH IMMINENT

↓

Request midwife if available
Prepare for newborn life support
Reassure the woman and support her in a comfortable position, avoiding the supine position
Provide Entonox for pain relief

↓

Support the birth of the baby's head by applying gentle pressure as head advances

↓

Support the baby during the birth and place on the maternal abdomen

↓

Thoroughly dry the baby with a warm towel and wrap with a dry towel

↓

If the baby is crying provide 'skin-to-skin' contact with the mother

→ If the baby is not crying refer to **Newborn Life Support**

↓

Allow the umbilical cord to stop pulsating prior to clamping and cutting

↓

The placenta may take 15–20 mins to birth – **DO NOT** pull on the cord – encourage the mother to pass urine

Deliver the placenta into a plastic bag for the midwife to inspect and check for completeness

Assess and record estimated blood loss

If the placenta remains undelivered with minimal bleeding, plan to transfer to the nearest appropriate destination as agreed locally

Maternal safety is the prime consideration

Consider the specific clinical situation **and which interventions may be required for the woman and baby on arrival**

Refer to 'Appropriate Destination for Conveyance' in **Maternity Care**

If the placenta remains undelivered and bleeding refer to Post-partum Haemorrhage

MATERNITY

Post-partum Haemorrhage

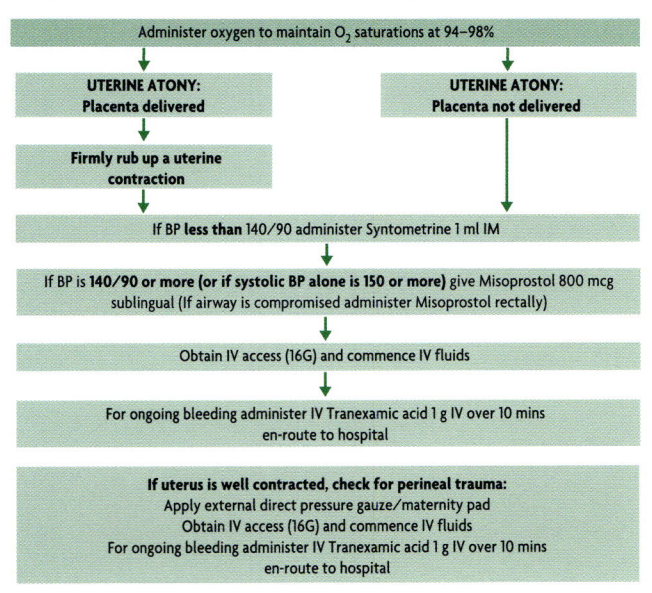

Administer oxygen to maintain O$_2$ saturations at 94–98%

| **UTERINE ATONY:** Placenta delivered | **UTERINE ATONY:** Placenta not delivered |

Firmly rub up a uterine contraction

If BP **less than** 140/90 administer Syntometrine 1 ml IM

If BP is **140/90 or more** (or if systolic BP alone is 150 or more) give Misoprostol 800 mcg sublingual (If airway is compromised administer Misoprostol rectally)

Obtain IV access (16G) and commence IV fluids

For ongoing bleeding administer IV Tranexamic acid 1 g IV over 10 mins en-route to hospital

If uterus is well contracted, check for perineal trauma:
Apply external direct pressure gauze/maternity pad
Obtain IV access (16G) and commence IV fluids
For ongoing bleeding administer IV Tranexamic acid 1 g IV over 10 mins
en-route to hospital

Transfer to nearest appropriate destination as agreed locally
Maternal safety is the prime consideration
Consider the specific clinical situation **and which interventions may be
required for the woman and baby on arrival**
Refer to 'Appropriate Destination for Conveyance' in **Maternity Care**
Pre-alert stating obstetric emergency PPH
Perform ongoing assessment of uterine contraction
and/or perineal trauma/maternal observations

Shoulder Dystocia

REQUEST A MIDWIFE IF AVAILABLE AND PREPARE FOR NEWBORN LIFE SUPPORT
Position the woman in the McRoberts position
For a solo clinician – ask the woman to hold her legs and push with her next contraction

↓

If shoulders do not release:
Attempt to deliver the baby
- With your hands on the baby's head apply gentle 'axial' traction, keeping the baby's head in line with its spine for up to 30 seconds

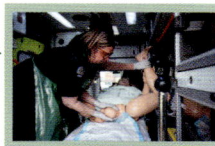

Undelivered?

Apply suprapubic pressure with the woman in the McRoberts position
- Identify the position of the fetal back and place assistant on that maternal side
- Using a CPR grip, apply continuous pressure downwards and lateral for 30 seconds (2 fingers above symphysis pubis)
- Encourage the woman to push **OR** attempt gentle 'axial' traction to deliver baby

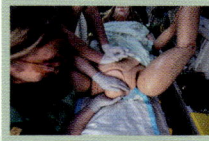

Undelivered?

- Attempt intermittent 'rocking' suprapubic pressure for 30 seconds and encourage woman to push
- Or attempt gentle 'axial' traction to deliver baby

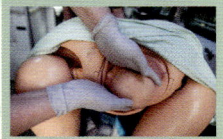

Undelivered?

- Change the woman's position to 'all fours' and encourage her to push
- Or attempt gentle 'axial' traction to deliver baby

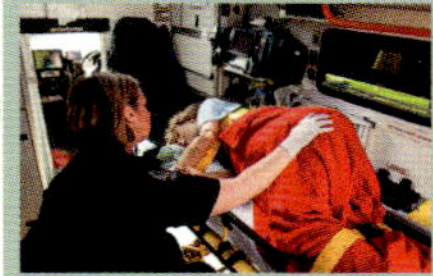

Undelivered?

- Walk the woman to the ambulance and anticipate the birth during transfer
- Convey in a lateral position with legs separated by a blanket to protect the baby's head
- Reassure the woman and provide Entonox as required.

Baby born
Refer to **Care of the Newborn**

75

MEDICINES

MEDS

Medicines: Best Practice Checklist

- Before administering any medication check the:
  - Type
  - Strength
  - Integrity of the packaging
  - Clarity of the fluid
  - Expiry date.
- Select the most appropriate route, taking into account:
  - The patient's condition
  - The urgency of the situation.
- Only administer drugs via the routes you have been trained for.
- The drug codes are provided for INFORMATION ONLY.
- Complete documentation.

Activated Charcoal ACT

Presentation
50 grams in 250 ml. Granules or suspension in water.

Indications
The emergency treatment of acute oral poisoning and oral drug overdose.

- Adults and children aged 1 and over who have ingested toxins less than 1 hour before attendance by an ambulance clinician.
  OR
- Adults and children, irrespective of time of ingestion, who have ingested toxins and where Toxbase or the National Poisons Information Service (0344 8920111) have been contacted and advised the administration of activated charcoal. **NB** Toxbase and the NPIS advice cannot overrule exclusion criteria except in relation to time and age.

Paracetamol overdose:

- The recommended dose of paracetamol is 4 g (or 75 mg/kg) in 24 hours for an adult patient.
- Any ingestion exceeding this is regarded as an overdose. However, toxicity is extremely unlikely if <75 mg/kg paracetamol has been ingested within a 24 hour period.
- Single acute overdose is defined as an ingestion of >4 g (or >75 mg/kg) in a period of <1 hour.
- The National Poisons Information Service (NPIS) in the UK recommends that, for the purposes of calculating potentially toxic doses, the following be considered:

79

see Medicines: Best Practice checklist **MEDS**

Activated Charcoal ACT

   a   For pregnant patients, the toxic dose is calculated using the patient's pre-pregnancy weight.

   b   For patients weighing >110 kg, the toxic dose should be calculated using a maximum of 110 kg instead of the patient's actual weight.

Contra-Indications

Children under 1 year.

Patients presenting to the ambulance clinician more than 1 hour since ingestion of toxin.

Administration not advised following communication from Toxbase or the NPIS.

Patients who are vomiting.

Patients with reduced gastro-intestinal motility (with a risk of obstruction), i.e. patients taking opioid medication or patients who have recently had abdominal surgery.

Poisoning known to be due to the ingestion of:

- Cyanide
- Petroleum distillates
- Metal salts including salts of lithium and iron
- Ethanol, methanol, ethylene glycol, iron salts, sodium chloride, lead boric acid, other mineral acid
- Malathion
- Corrosive substances (limited usefulness and hinders the visualisation of oesophageal burns or erosions).

Activated Charcoal ACT

Cautions

Precautions should be taken to prevent aspiration, especially in small children.

Activated charcoal will reduce the effectiveness of other antidotes.

Patients who have taken an overdose and have also consumed recreational alcohol can be administered activated charcoal providing that they are alert enough to safely swallow the charcoal.

Shake the bottle vigorously before administration.

Side Effects

Black stools.

Intestinal obstruction (blockage of digestive system).

Bezoar formation (ball of material in the stomach that is not passed out).

Intestinal perforation (rare, but can occur after several treatments).

Dosage and Administration

Administer as soon as possible after ingestion or suspected ingestion of the potential poison.

For adults, give a single dose of 50 grams (250 ml) of activated charcoal, as soon as possible after ingestion or suspected ingestion of the potential poison.

*see Medicines: Best Practice checklist **MEDS**

Activated Charcoal   ACT

For children aged 1 year to under 12 years, encourage the child to drink 125 ml, equivalent to 25 grams of activated charcoal or half of the contents of one bottle, unless a large quantity of poison has been ingested, and where there is a risk to life. In these circumstances, the administration of the full 50 grams dose is indicated.

May be mixed with soft drinks or fruit juice to mask the flavour. However, ice cream or other foods should not be used as a vehicle for the administration of activated charcoal as they reduce the adsorptive capacity of the activated charcoal.

Route: Oral

AGE	INITIAL DOSE	REPEAT DOSE	DOSE INTERVAL	VOLUME	MAXIMUM DOSE
≥ 12 years 50 grams in 250 ml	50 g	N/A	N/A	250 ml	50 grams

NOTE: Concentration is only applicable to ready-made suspension.

Adrenaline 1 milligram in 10 ml (1 in 10,000) ADX

Presentation

Pre-filled syringe containing 1 milligram of adrenaline (epinephrine) in 10 ml (1:10,000) ADX.

Indications

Cardiac arrest.

Actions

Adrenaline is a sympathomimetic that stimulates both alpha- and beta-adrenergic receptors. As a result myocardial and cerebral blood flow is enhanced during CPR and CPR becomes more effective due to increased peripheral resistance which improves perfusion pressures.

*see Medicines: Best Practice checklist**MEDS**

Adrenaline 1 milligram in 10 ml (1 in 10,000)   ADX

Cautions

Severe hypertension may occur in patients on non-cardioselective beta-blockers (e.g. Propranolol).

Do **NOT** administer adrenaline when the patient's core temperature is less than 30°C. When the patient's temperature is between 30°C and 35°C, double the time period between doses.

Dosage and Administration

Cardiac arrest:

- **Shockable rhythms:** administer adrenaline after the 3rd shock and then after alternate shocks (i.e. 5th, 7th etc).

- **Non-shockable rhythms:** administer adrenaline immediately IV access is achieved then alternate loops.

Route: Intravenous/intraosseous – **administer as a rapid bolus**.

AGE	INITIAL DOSE	REPEAT DOSE	DOSE INTERVAL	VOLUME	MAXIMUM DOSE
≥12 years and Adult 1 milligram in 10 ml (1:10,000)	1 milligram	1 milligram	3–5 minutes	10 ml	No limit

Adrenaline 1 milligram in 1 ml (1 in 1,000) ADM

Presentation
Pre-filled syringe or ampoule containing 1 milligram of adrenaline (epinephrine) in 1 ml (1:1,000) ADM.

Indications
Anaphylaxis.

Life-threatening asthma with failing ventilation and continued deterioration despite nebuliser therapy.

Actions
Adrenaline is a sympathomimetic that stimulates both alpha- and beta-adrenergic receptors. As a result myocardial and cerebral blood flow is enhanced during CPR and CPR becomes more effective due to increased peripheral resistance which improves perfusion pressures.

Reverses allergic manifestations of acute anaphylaxis.

Relieves bronchospasm in acute severe asthma.

Cautions
Severe hypertension may occur in patients on non-cardioselective beta-blockers (e.g. Propranolol).

Do **NOT** administer IV adrenaline in cases of anaphylaxis.

see Medicines: Best Practice checklist **MEDS**

Adrenaline 1 milligram in 1 ml (1 in 1,000)

ADM

Dosage and Administration

Intramuscular
Anaphylaxis and **life-threatening asthma.**
Route: Intramuscular – antero-lateral aspect of thigh.

AGE	INITIAL DOSE	REPEAT DOSE	DOSE INTERVAL	VOLUME	MAX DOSE
≥12 years and adult 1 milligram in 1 ml (1:1,000)	500 micrograms	500 micrograms	5 minutes	0.5 ml	No limit

Amiodarone Hydrochloride   AMO

Presentation
Pre-filled syringe containing 300 milligrams amiodarone in 10 ml.

Indications
Cardiac arrest
- **Shockable rhythms:** if unresponsive to defibrillation administer amiodarone after the 3rd shock and an additional bolus depending on age to unresponsive VF or pulseless VT following the 5th shock.

Actions
Antiarrhythmic; lengthens cardiac action potential and therefore effective refractory period. Prolongs QT interval on ECG.

Blocks sodium and potassium channels in cardiac muscle.

Acts to stabilise and reduce electrical irritability of cardiac muscle.

Contra-Indications
No contra-indications in the context of the treatment of cardiac arrest.

Side Effects
Bradycardia.

Vasodilatation causing hypotension, flushing.

Bronchospasm.

Arrhythmias – Torsades de pointes.

*see Medicines: Best Practice checklist   **MEDS**

Amiodarone Hydrochloride   AMO

Dosage and Administration

- Administer into large vein as extravasation can cause burns.
- Follow administration with a 0.9% sodium chloride flush – **refer to Sodium Chloride**.
- Cardiac arrest – Shockable rhythms: if unresponsive to defibrillation administer amiodarone after the 3rd shock.

Route: intravenous/intraosseous – administer as a rapid bolus.

AGE	INITIAL DOSE	REPEAT DOSE	DOSE INTERVAL	VOLUME	MAXIMUM DOSE
Adult 300 milligrams in 10 ml	300 milligrams (After 3rd shock)	150 milligrams	After 5th shock	10 ml	450 milligrams

Aspirin ASP

Presentation

300 milligrams aspirin (acetylsalicylic acid) in tablet form. Dispersible or chewable.

Indications

Adults with:

- Clinical or ECG evidence suggestive of myocardial infarction or ischaemia.

Actions

Has an antiplatelet action which reduces clot formation.

Contra-indications

- Known aspirin allergy or sensitivity.
- Children under 16 years (see additional information).
- Active gastrointestinal bleeding.
- Haemophilia or other known clotting disorders.
- Severe hepatic failure with jaundice.

Cautions

As the likely benefits of a single 300 milligram aspirin outweigh the potential risks, aspirin may be given to patients with:

- Asthma
- Pregnancy

*see Medicines: Best Practice checklist   **MEDS**

Aspirin   ASP

- Renal failure
- Moderate hepatic disease without jaundice
- Gastric or duodenal ulcer
- Current treatment with anticoagulants.

Side Effects
- Increased risk of gastric bleeding.
- Wheezing in some asthmatics.

Additional Information

In suspected myocardial infarction a 300 milligram aspirin tablet should be given regardless of any previous aspirin taken that day.

Clopidogrel may be indicated in acute ST segment elevation myocardial infarction – refer to **Clopidogrel**.

Aspirin is contra-indicated in children under the age of 16 years as it may precipitate Reye's syndrome. This syndrome is very rare and occurs in young children, damaging the liver and brain. It has a mortality rate of 50%.

Dosage and Administration

Route: Oral – chewed or dissolved in water.

AGE	INITIAL DOSE	REPEAT DOSE	DOSE INTERVAL	VOLUME	MAX DOSE
Adults 300 milligrams per tablet	300 milligrams	NONE	N/A	1 tablet	300 milligrams

Atropine Sulfate — ATR

Presentation

Pre-filled syringe containing 1 milligram atropine sulfate in 10 ml (100 microgram atropine sulfate per 1 ml).

Pre-filled syringe containing 1 milligram atropine sulfate in 5 ml (200 microgram atropine sulfate per 1 ml).

Pre-filled syringe containing 3 milligrams atropine sulfate in 10 ml (300 microgram atropine sulfate per 1 ml).

An ampoule containing 600 micrograms in 1 ml.

Indications

Symptomatic bradycardia in the presence of **ANY** of these adverse signs:

- Absolute bradycardia (pulse <40 beats per minute).
- Systolic blood pressure below expected for age (refer to **Page-for-Age** for age related blood pressure readings in children).
- Paroxysmal ventricular arrhythmias requiring suppression.
- Inadequate perfusion causing confusion, etc.
- Bradycardia following return of spontaneous circulation (ROSC).

NB Hypoxia is the most common cause of bradycardia in children, therefore interventions to support ABC and oxygen therapy should be the first-line therapy.

Refer also to **Atropine for CBRNE**.

Contra-indications

Should **NOT** be given to treat bradycardia in suspected hypothermia.

*see Medicines: Best Practice checklist **MEDS**

Atropine Sulfate　　　　　　　**ATR**

Actions

Reverses effects of vagal overdrive.

Increases heart rate by blocking vagal activity in sinus bradycardia, second or third degree heart block.

Enhances A-V conduction.

Side Effects

Dry mouth, visual blurring and pupil dilation.

Confusion and occasional hallucinations.

Tachycardia.

Do not use small (<100 micrograms) doses as they may cause paradoxical bradycardia.

Additional Information

May induce tachycardia when used after myocardial infarction, which will increase myocardial oxygen demand and worsen ischaemia. Hence, bradycardia in a patient with an MI should **ONLY** be treated if the low heart rate is causing problems with perfusion.

May not improve bradycardia in patients who have had a heart transplant.

Atropine Sulfate — ATR

Dosage and Administration

SYMPTOMATIC BRADYCARDIA

NB BRADYCARDIA in children is most commonly caused by **HYPOXIA**, requiring immediate ABC care, **NOT** drug therapy; therefore **ONLY** administer atropine in cases of bradycardia caused by vagal stimulation (e.g. suction).

Route: Intravenous/intraosseous **administer as a rapid bolus**.

AGE	INITIAL DOSE	REPEAT DOSE	DOSE INTERVAL	VOLUME	MAX DOSE
≥12 years 600 micrograms per ml	600 micrograms*	600 micrograms*	3–5 minutes	1 ml	3 milligrams

Route: Intravenous/intraosseous **administer as a rapid bolus**.

AGE	INITIAL DOSE	REPEAT DOSE	DOSE INTERVAL	VOLUME	MAX DOSE
≥12 years 300 micrograms per ml	600 micrograms*	600 micrograms*	3–5 minutes	2 ml	3 milligrams

*The adult dosage can be given as 500 or 600 micrograms to a maximum of 3 milligrams depending on presentation available.

*see Medicines: Best Practice checklist **MEDS**

Atropine Sulfate   ATR

Route: Intravenous/intraosseous **administer as a rapid bolus**.

AGE	INITIAL DOSE	REPEAT DOSE	DOSE INTERVAL	VOLUME	MAX DOSE
≥12 years 200 micrograms per ml	600 micrograms*	600 micrograms*	3–5 minutes	3 ml	3 milligrams

Route: Intravenous/intraosseous **administer as a rapid bolus**.

AGE	INITIAL DOSE	REPEAT DOSE	DOSE INTERVAL	VOLUME	MAX DOSE
≥12 years 100 micrograms per ml	600 micrograms*	600 micrograms*	3–5 minutes	6 ml	3 milligrams

*The adult dosage can be given as 500 or 600 micrograms to a maximum of 3 milligrams depending on presentation available.

Benzylpenicillin Sodium BPN

Presentation

Injection vial containing 600 milligrams of benzylpenicillin sodium as powder for solution for injection.

Injection vial containing 1.2 gram of benzylpenicillin sodium powder for solution for injection.

Administered intravenously, intraosseously or intramuscularly.

NB Different concentrations and volumes of administration (**refer to dosage and administration tables**).

Indications

Suspected meningococcal disease in the presence of:

1 a non-blanching rash (the classical, haemorrhagic, non-blanching rash (may be petechial or purpuric)

and/or

2 signs/symptoms suggestive of meningococcal septicaemia (**refer to Meningococcal Meningitis and Septicaemia for signs/symptoms**).

Actions

Antibiotic: narrow-spectrum.

Contra-Indications

Known severe penicillin allergy (more than a simple rash alone).

Additional Information

- Meningococcal septicaemia is commonest in children and young adults.

see Medicines: Best Practice checklist **MEDS**

Benzylpenicillin Sodium   **BPN**

- It may be rapidly progressive and fatal.
- Early administration of benzylpenicillin improves outcome.
- Two sites should be used for IM injection when administering more than 2ml of volume.

Dosage and Administration

Administer en-route to hospital (unless already administered).

NB IV/IO and IM concentrations are different and have different volumes of administration.

Route: Intravenous/intraosseous — by slow injection.

AGE	INITIAL DOSE	REPEAT DOSE	DOSE INTERVAL	VOLUME	MAXIMUM DOSE
Adult 1.2 grams dissolved in 20 ml water for injection	1.2 grams	NONE	N/A	20 ml	1.2 grams

Route: Intramuscular (antero-lateral aspect of thigh or upper arm — preferably in a well perfused area) if rapid intravascular access cannot be obtained.

AGE	INITIAL DOSE	REPEAT DOSE	DOSE INTERVAL	VOLUME	MAXIMUM DOSE
Adult 1.2 grams dissolved in 4 ml water for injection	1.2 grams	NONE	N/A	4 ml	1.2 grams

Chlorphenamine CPH

Presentation
Ampoule containing 10 milligrams of chlorphenamine maleate in 1 ml.

Tablet containing 4 milligrams of chlorphenamine maleate.

Oral solution containing 2 milligrams of chlorphenamine maleate in 5 ml.

Indications
Severe anaphylactic reactions after initial resuscitation.

Symptomatic allergic reactions falling short of anaphylaxis but causing patient distress (e.g. severe itching).

Actions
An antihistamine with anticholingergic properties that blocks the effect of histamine released during a hypersensitivity (allergic) reaction.

Contra-Indications
Known hypersensitivity.

The anticholinergic properties of chlorphenamine are intensified by monoamine oxidase inhibitors (MAOIs). Chlorphenamine injection is therefore contraindicated in patients who have been treated with MAOIs within the last fourteen days.

Cautions
Pregnancy and breastfeeding.

Hypotension.

*see Medicines: Best Practice checklist **MEDS**

Chlorphenamine   **CPH**

Epilepsy.

Glaucoma.

Severe liver disease.

Side Effects

Sedation.

Dry mouth.

Headache.

Blurred vision.

Urinary retention.

Psychomotor impairment.

Gastrointestinal disturbance.

Convulsions (rare).

Children and older people are more likely to suffer side effects.

Warn anyone receiving chlorphenamine against driving or undertaking any other complex psychomotor task, due to the sedative and psychomotor side effects.

With the intravenous preparation, transient hypotension, central nervous system (CNS) stimulation and irritant effects.

Chlorphenamine   CPH

Dosage and Administration

Route: Intravenous/intraosseous/intramuscular. The IV route is the preferred route for anaphylaxis, given SLOWLY over 1 minute. Small doses can be diluted with sodium chloride 0.9%.

AGE	INITIAL DOSE	REPEAT DOSE	DOSE INTERVAL	VOLUME	MAXIMUM DOSE
≥12 years 10 milligrams in 1 ml	10 milligrams	NONE	N/A	1 ml	10 milligrams

Route: Oral 4 milligram tablet.

AGE	INITIAL DOSE	REPEAT DOSE	DOSE INTERVAL	VOLUME	MAXIMUM DOSE
≥12 years 4 milligrams per tablet	4 milligrams	NONE	N/A	1 tablet	4 milligrams

Route: Oral 2 milligrams in 5 ml solution.

AGE	INITIAL DOSE	REPEAT DOSE	DOSE INTERVAL	VOLUME	MAXIMUM DOSE
≥12 years 2 milligrams in 5 ml	4 milligrams	NONE	N/A	10 ml	4 milligrams

*see Medicines: Best Practice checklist | **MEDS**

Clopidogrel   **CLO**

Presentation

Tablet containing clopidogrel:

- 75 milligrams
- 300 milligrams.

Indications

Acute ST-elevation myocardial infarction (STEMI):

- In patients not already taking clopidogrel.
- In patients receiving thrombolytic treatment.
- Anticipated thrombolytic treatment.
- Anticipated primary percutaneous coronary intervention (PPCI).

Actions

Inhibits platelet aggregation.

Contra-Indications

- Known allergy or hypersensitivity to clopidogrel.
- Known severe liver impairment.
- Active pathological bleeding such as peptic ulcer or intracranial haemorrhage.

Cautions

As the likely benefits of a single dose of clopidogrel outweigh the potential risks, clopidogrel may be administered in:

- Pregnancy.

Clopidogrel CLO

- Patients taking non-steroidal anti-inflammatory drugs (NSAIDs).
- Patients with renal impairment.

Side Effects

- Dyspepsia.
- Abdominal pain.
- Diarrhoea.
- Bleeding (gastrointestinal and intracranial) – the occurrence of severe bleeding is similar to that observed with the administration of aspirin.

Dosage and Administration

Adults aged 18–75 years with acute ST-elevation myocardial infarction (STEMI) receiving thrombolysis or anticipated primary PCI, as per locally agreed STEMI care pathways.

NOTE: To be administered in conjunction with aspirin unless there is a known aspirin allergy or sensitivity (**refer to Aspirin for administration and dosage**).

*see Medicines: Best Practice checklist   **MEDS**

Clopidogrel   CLO

Route: Oral.

Patient care pathway: Thrombolysis.

AGE	INITIAL DOSE	REPEAT DOSE	DOSE INTERVAL	VOLUME	MAXIMUM DOSE
Adult 300 milligrams per tablet	300 milligrams	NONE	N/A	1 tablet	300 milligrams
Adult 75 milligrams per tablet	300 milligrams	NONE	N/A	4 tablets	300 milligrams

Patient care pathway: Primary percutaneous coronary intervention.

AGE	INITIAL DOSE	REPEAT DOSE	DOSE INTERVAL	VOLUME	MAXIMUM DOSE
Adult 300 milligrams per tablet	600 milligrams	NONE	N/A	2 tablets	600 milligrams
Adult 75 milligrams per tablet	600 milligrams	NONE	N/A	8 tablets	600 milligrams

Dexamethasone — DEX

Presentation
- Dexamethasone 2 milligrams in 5 ml oral solution, sugar free
- Dexamethasone 2 milligram soluble tablets, sugar free

Where the oral solution, which is licensed to treat croup in children, is available this should be used to provide the most accurate dose.

Indications
Mild/moderate/severe croup, scored using the Modified Taussig Score, refer to **Respiratory Illness in Children**.

Actions
Corticosteroid – reduces subglottic inflammation.

Contra-indications
Impending respiratory failure.

Cautions
Upper airway compromise can be worsened by any procedure that distresses the child – this might include the administration of medication.

Side Effects
- Gastro-intestinal upset.
- Hypersensitivity/anaphylactic reaction.

*see Medicines: Best Practice checklist   **MEDS**

Dexamethasone   DEX

Additional Information

A single pre-hospital dose is advised. If you feel the child needs a second dose in the same episode of illness they must be reviewed by a senior healthcare professional; seek senior clinical advice.

If the child vomits less than 30 minutes after administration, the same dose can be given again.

Dosage and Administration

Route: Oral solution. The doses given in the following dosage chart are taken from the Summary of Product Characteristics of the oral solution licensed for use in childhood croup. The doses are calculated on average weights to give a dose of dexamethasone of 0.15mg/kg.

AGE	INITIAL DOSE	REPEAT DOSE	DOSE INTERVAL	VOLUME	MAX DOSE
11 years 2 milligrams in 5 ml	6 milligrams	NONE	N/A	15 ml	6 milligrams
10 years 2 milligrams in 5 ml	6 milligrams	NONE	N/A	15 ml	6 milligrams
9 years 2 milligrams in 5 ml	6 milligrams	NONE	N/A	15 ml	6 milligrams
8 years 2 milligrams in 5 ml	4 milligrams	NONE	N/A	10 ml	4 milligrams

Dexamethasone — DEX

AGE	INITIAL DOSE	REPEAT DOSE	DOSE INTERVAL	VOLUME	MAX DOSE
7 years 2 milligrams in 5 ml	4 milligrams	NONE	N/A	10 ml	4 milligrams
6 years 2 milligrams in 5 ml	3.2 milligrams	NONE	N/A	8 ml	3.2 milligrams
5 years 2 milligrams in 5 ml	3.2 milligrams	NONE	N/A	8 ml	3.2 milligrams
4 years 2 milligrams in 5 ml	3.2 milligrams	NONE	N/A	8 ml	3.2 milligrams
3 years 2 milligrams in 5 ml	2.4 milligrams	NONE	N/A	6 ml	2.4 milligrams
2 years 2 milligrams in 5 ml	2 milligrams	NONE	N/A	5 ml	2 milligrams
18 months 2 milligrams in 5 ml	2 milligrams	NONE	N/A	5 ml	2 milligrams
12 months 2 milligrams in 5 ml	2 milligrams	NONE	N/A	5 ml	2 milligrams

*see Medicines: Best Practice checklist   **MEDS**

Dexamethasone   **DEX**

AGE	INITIAL DOSE	REPEAT DOSE	DOSE INTERVAL	VOLUME	MAX DOSE
9 months 2 milligrams in 5 ml	1.6 milligram	NONE	N/A	4 ml	1.6 milligram
6 months 2 milligrams in 5 ml	1.6 milligram	NONE	N/A	4 ml	1.6 milligram
3 months 2 milligrams in 5 ml	1.2 milligram	NONE	N/A	3 ml	1.2 milligram
1 month 2 milligrams in 5 ml	0.8 milligram	NONE	N/A	2 ml	0.8 milligram
Birth	N/A	N/A	N/A	N/A	N/A

Route: Oral tablet. Dissolve the 2 milligram tablets in water.

AGE	INITIAL DOSE	REPEAT DOSE	DOSE INTERVAL	VOLUME	MAX DOSE
11 years 2 milligrams per tablet	6 milligrams	NONE	N/A	3 tablets	6 milligrams
10 years 2 milligrams per tablet	6 milligrams	NONE	N/A	3 tablets	6 milligrams
9 years 2 milligrams per tablet	6 milligrams	NONE	N/A	3 tablets	6 milligrams

Dexamethasone — DEX

AGE	INITIAL DOSE	REPEAT DOSE	DOSE INTERVAL	VOLUME	MAX DOSE
8 years 2 milligrams per tablet	4 milligrams	NONE	N/A	2 tablets	4 milligrams
7 years 2 milligrams per tablet	4 milligrams	NONE	N/A	2 tablets	4 milligrams
6 years 2 milligrams per tablet	4 milligrams	NONE	N/A	2 tablets	4 milligrams
5 years 2 milligrams per tablet	4 milligrams	NONE	N/A	2 tablets	4 milligrams
4 years 2 milligrams per tablet	4 milligrams	NONE	N/A	2 tablets	4 milligrams
3 years 2 milligrams per tablet	2 milligrams	NONE	N/A	1 tablet	2 milligrams
2 years 2 milligrams per tablet	2 milligrams	NONE	N/A	1 tablet	2 milligrams
18 months 2 milligrams per tablet	2 milligrams	NONE	N/A	1 tablet	2 milligrams

*see Medicines: Best Practice checklist **MEDS**

Dexamethasone   **DEX**

AGE	INITIAL DOSE	REPEAT DOSE	DOSE INTERVAL	VOLUME	MAX DOSE
12 months 2 milligrams per tablet	2 milligrams	NONE	N/A	1 tablet	2 milligrams
9 months 2 milligrams per tablet	2 milligrams	NONE	N/A	1 tablet	2 milligrams
6 months 2 milligrams per tablet	2 milligrams	NONE	N/A	1 tablet	2 milligrams
3 months 2 milligrams per tablet	2 milligrams	NONE	N/A	1 tablet	2 milligrams
1 month 2 milligrams per tablet	2 milligrams	NONE	N/A	1 tablet	2 milligrams
Birth	N/A	N/A	N/A	N/A	N/A

Diazepam   DZP

Presentation

Ampoule containing 10 milligrams diazepam in an oil-in-water emulsion making up 2 ml.

Diazepam 10mg/2ml solution for injection (only used when the emulsion is unavailable as more irritant than emulsion).

Rectal tube containing 2.5 milligrams, 5 milligrams or 10 milligrams diazepam.

Indications

Patients who have prolonged convulsions (lasting 5 minutes or more) **OR** repeated convulsions (three or more in an hour), and are **CURRENTLY CONVULSING** – not secondary to an uncorrected hypoxic or hypoglycaemic episode (see 'Additional Information' below).

Eclamptic convulsions (initiate treatment if seizure lasts over 2–3 minutes or if it is recurrent).

Symptomatic cocaine toxicity (severe hypertension, chest pain or convulsions).

Actions

Central nervous system depressant, acts as an anticonvulsant and sedative.

Cautions

Should be used with caution if alcohol, antidepressants or other CNS depressants have been taken as side effects are more likely.

*see Medicines: Best Practice checklist **MEDS**

Diazepam   DZP

A dose of buccal midazolam or rectal diazepam given by a parent or carer may be the first dose administered for this seizure. The first dose given by the paramedic may be the second dose of benzodiazepine given for the seizure and IV/IO access may be needed, refer to **Convulsions in Adults**.

Contra-indications

Patients with known hypersensitivity.

Side Effects

Respiratory depression may occur, especially in the presence of alcohol (which enhances the depressive side effect of diazepam). Opioid drugs similarly enhance diazepam's cardiac and respiratory depressive effects.

Hypotension may occur. This may be significant if the patient has to be moved from a horizontal position to allow for extrication from an address. Caution should therefore be exercised and consideration given to either removing the patient flat or, if the convulsion has stopped and it is considered safe, allowing a 10-minute recovery period prior to removal.

Other side effects include light-headedness, unsteadiness, drowsiness, confusion and amnesia.

Additional Information

If the patient is prescribed buccal midazolam and a supply is available, this may be administered according to the prescriber's instructions.

Diazepam DZP

Diazepam should only be used if the patient has been convulsing for 5 minutes or more, or if convulsions recur in rapid succession without time for full recovery in between (and in either case is <u>still convulsing</u>). There is no value in giving 'preventative' diazepam if the convulsion has ceased.

In any clearly sick or ill child, there must be no delay at the scene while administering the drug – it can be administered en-route to hospital.

If IV access can be gained rapidly, then this is preferable to the PR route. If buccal midazolam is available, use that in preference to gaining IV access for the first dose of diazepam.

Early consideration should be given to using the buccal or PR route when IV access cannot be rapidly and safely obtained, **commonly the case in children**. In small children the buccal or PR route should be considered the first treatment option (with IV access being sought subsequently). When giving rectal medication, offer parental explanation and maintain patient dignity.

All patients who continue to convulse should receive a total of **TWO** doses of benzodiazepine (midazolam or diazepam) 10 minutes apart, the second dose should be IV/IO if possible. Only give a second rectal dose if IV/IO access cannot be obtained in the 10 minutes between the first and second doses. Seek clinical advice if the convulsion continues 10 minutes after the second dose.

Care must be taken when inserting rectal tubes. They should be inserted no more than 2.5 cm in children or 4–5 cm in adults. All tubes have an insertion marker on the nozzle.

*see Medicines: Best Practice checklist **MEDS**

Diazepam   DZP

The **full** dose should be given at the appropriate times. It is **not** appropriate to either i) gradually 'titrate the dose upwards' or ii) to only give a partial dose if the convulsion stops (once started, even if the convulsion stops, that dose must be given). If this approach is followed, convulsion recurrence is much less likely.

Dosage and Administration

Route: Rectal

For convulsions give the full dose.

*NB In recurrent or ongoing convulsions, for the second dose, IV/IO access is recommended.

AGE	INITIAL DOSE	REPEAT DOSE*	DOSE INTERVAL	VOLUME	MAX DOSE
Adult ≥70 years 10 milligrams in 2.5 ml	10 milligrams	10 milligrams	10 minutes	1 x 10 milligram tube	20 milligrams
Adult <70 years 10 milligrams in 2.5 ml	20 milligrams	10 milligrams	10 minutes	1 or 2 x 10 milligram tube	30 milligrams

Diazepam — DZP

Route: Intravenous/intraosseous – administer **SLOWLY** over 2 minutes for adults (3–5 minutes for children).

For convulsions give the full dose. In symptomatic cocaine toxicity titrate slowly to response.

NB The second benzodiazepine dose should be IV/IO wherever possible (i.e. IV/IO diazepam).

Where a first adult <70 years dose of 20 milligrams diazepam has been given rectally and the patient continues to fit, a second dose of 10 milligrams diazepam should be administered IV, giving a total cumulative dose of 30 milligrams diazepam. Where both first and second doses are given IV then the maximum cumulative dose is 20 milligrams.

Be ready to support ventilations.

AGE	INITIAL DOSE	REPEAT DOSE	DOSE INTERVAL	VOLUME	MAX DOSE
Adult 10 milligrams in 2 ml	10 milligrams	10 milligrams	10 minutes	2 ml	20 milligrams

*see Medicines: Best Practice checklist **MEDS**

Furosemide   FRM

Presentation
20 milligrams in 2 ml injection ampoules
50 milligrams in 5 ml injection ampoules

Indications
Consider IV furosemide for pulmonary oedema due to acute heart failure.

Actions
Furosemide is a potent diuretic with a rapid onset (within 30 minutes) and short duration.

Contra-Indications
- Reduced GCS with liver cirrhosis.
- Cardiogenic shock.
- Severe renal failure with anuria.
- Children under 18 years old.

Cautions
Hypokalaemia (low potassium) could induce arrhythmias.

Pregnancy.

Hypotensive patient.

Furosemide FRM

Side Effects
Hypotension.

Gastrointestinal disturbances.

Additional Information
Consider furosemide when the time to get the patient to hospital is prolonged.

Dosage and Administration
Route: Intravenous – administer **SLOWLY OVER** 2 minutes in accordance with the table below.

AGE	INITIAL DOSE	REPEAT DOSE	DOSE INTERVAL	VOLUME	MAXIMUM DOSE
Adult 18 years and over 20 milligrams/2 ml	40 milligrams	NONE	N/A	4 ml	40 milligrams
Adult 18 years and over 50 milligrams/5 ml	40 milligrams	NONE	N/A	4 ml	40 milligrams

see Medicines: Best Practice checklist **MEDS**

Glucagon   GLU

Presentation

Glucagon injection, 1 milligram of powder in vial for reconstitution with water for injection.

Indications

Hypoglycaemia, clinically suspected hypoglycaemia or unconscious patients where hypoglycaemia is considered a likely cause (blood glucose <4.0 millimoles per litre).

NB Glucagon should only be administered when oral glucose administration is not possible or is ineffective, **AND/OR** when IV access to administer 10% glucose is not possible.

Actions

Glucagon is a hormone that induces the conversion of glycogen to glucose in the liver, thereby raising blood glucose levels.

Contra-Indications

- Pheochromocytoma.
- Glucagon should NOT be given by IV injection because of increased vomiting associated with IV use.

Cautions

- Low glycogen stores (e.g. recent use of glucagon or starvation).
- For hypoglycaemic seizures, glucose 10% IV is the preferred intervention.

Glucagon GLU

Side Effects
- Nausea, vomiting.
- Abdominal pain in adults.
- Diarrhoea in children.
- Hypokalaemia.
- Hypotension in adults.
- Acute hypersensitivity reaction, although this is rare.

Additional Information
- Check whether glucagon has already been administered by a relative/carer.
- Glucagon should only be administered once.
- Confirm effectiveness by checking blood glucose 10 to 15 minutes after administration.
- Glucagon may take up to 15 minutes to work.
- Glucagon can be ineffective in the very young, older people, undernourished patients or those with hepatic disease. Glucagon is relatively ineffective once body glycogen stores have been exhausted, especially in hypoglycaemic, non-diabetic children.
- When treating hypoglycaemia, use all available clinical information to help decide between glucagon IM, glucose 40% oral gel, or glucose 10% IV.

see Medicines: Best Practice checklist **MEDS**

Glucagon   GLU

- Hypoglycaemic patients who are convulsing should preferably be given glucose 10% IV.
  - If the patient is conscious, use glucose 40% gel as first line treatment. Unconscious patients will require glucose 10% IV.
  - A newborn baby's liver has very limited glycogen stores, so hypoglycaemia may not be effectively treated using intramuscular glucagon. Glucagon works by stimulating the liver to convert glycogen into glucose.
  - Glucagon may also be ineffective in some instances of alcohol-induced hypoglycaemia.

Dosage and Administration

Route: Intramuscular – antero-lateral aspect of thigh or upper arm.

AGE	INITIAL DOSE	REPEAT DOSE	DOSE INTERVAL	VOLUME	MAXIMUM DOSE
Adult ≥12 years 1 milligram per vial	1 milligram	NONE	N/A	1 vial	1 milligram

NB If no response within 10 minutes, administer intravenous glucose – **refer to Glucose 10%**.

Glucose 10%   GLX

Presentation
500 ml pack of 10% glucose solution (50 grams).

WARNING! Glucose and saline fluid bags are commonly confused as they are both clear fluids. STOP and CHECK before administration.

Indications
Hypoglycaemia (blood glucose <4.0 millimoles per litre) or suspected hypoglycaemia when oral administration is not possible and a rapid improvement in clinical state and blood glucose level is required.

An unconscious patient, where hypoglycaemia is considered a likely cause.

Management of hypoglycaemia in patients who have not responded to the administration of IM Glucagon after 10 minutes.

Actions
Reversal of hypoglycaemia by direct delivery of glucose (sugar) to the systemic circulation.

Cautions
Flush IV line thoroughly with sodium chloride 0.9% after administration to reduce vein irritation from residual glucose injection, refer to **0.9% Sodium Chloride**.

Contra-indications
IM or subcutaneous injection.

*see Medicines: Best Practice checklist | MEDS

Glucose 10% GLX

Additional Information

When treating hypoglycaemia, use all available clinical information to help decide between Glucose 10% IV, Glucose 40% oral gel, or Glucagon IM.

The IO route of administration may be used in exceptional cases when IV access cannot be obtained and other methods are not possible/effective. There is an increased risk of osteomyelitis compared to isotonic fluids.

Dosage and Administration

IV infusion: Peripherally via secure cannula into large vein or central access as Glucose 10% is an irritant, especially if extravasation occurs.

If the patient has shown no response, the dose may be repeated after 5 minutes.

If the patient has shown a **PARTIAL** response then a further infusion may be necessary, titrated to response to restore a normal GCS.

If after the second dose there has been **NO** response, pre-alert and transport rapidly to further care. Consider an alternative diagnosis or the likelihood of a third dose en-route benefiting the patient.

Glucose 10%   GLX

Intravenous/intraosseous infusion

Route: Intravenous/intraosseous infusion.

NB Neonatal doses are intentionally larger per kilo than those used in older children.

AGE	INITIAL DOSE	REPEAT DOSE	DOSE INTERVAL	VOLUME	MAXIMUM DOSE
Adult ≥12 years 50 grams in 500 ml	10 grams glucose	10 grams glucose	5 minutes	100 ml	300 ml (30 g glucose)

*see Medicines: Best Practice checklist   MEDS

Glucose 40% Oral Gel   GLG

Presentation
Plastic tube containing 25g glucose 40% oral gel.

Indications
Known or suspected hypoglycaemia in a conscious patient where there is no risk of choking or aspiration.

Actions
Rapid increase in blood glucose levels via buccal absorption.

Cautions
Altered consciousness – risk of choking or aspiration (in such circumstances glucose gel can be administered by soaking a gauze swab and placing it between the patient's lip and gum to aid absorption).

Side Effects
None.

Additional Information
Can be repeated as necessary in the hypoglycaemic patient.

Treatment failure should prompt the use of an alternative such as glucagon IM or glucose 10% IV.

(**Refer to Glucagon or Glucose 10%**).

Contra-Indications
None.

Glucose 40% Oral Gel — GLG

Dosage and Administration

Route: Buccal – Measure blood glucose level after each dose.

The gel should be squeezed into the mouth between the teeth and gums.

AGE	INITIAL DOSE	REPEAT DOSE	DOSE INTERVAL	VOLUME	MAXIMUM DOSE
Adults ≥ 12 years 10 grams in 25 grams of gel	10–20 grams	10 grams	5 minutes	1–2 tubes	2 tubes/ 20grams

NB Assess more frequently in children who require a smaller dose for a response. This medicine should only be administered if the child has a gag reflex.

NB Consider IM glucagon or IV glucose 10% if no clinical improvement.

*see Medicines: Best Practice checklist

MEDS

Glyceryl Trinitrate (GTN) **GTN**

Presentation

Sublingual spray containing 400 micrograms glyceryl trinitrate per metered dose.

Sublingual tablets containing glyceryl trinitrate 300, 500 or 600 micrograms per tablet.

Indications

Cardiac chest pain due to angina or myocardial infarction, when systolic blood pressure is greater than 90mmHg.

Breathlessness due to pulmonary oedema in acute heart failure when systolic blood pressure is greater than 110 mmHg.

Patients with suspected cocaine toxicity presenting with chest pain.

Actions

A potent vasodilator drug resulting in:

- Dilatation of coronary arteries/relief of coronary spasm.
- Dilatation of systemic veins resulting in lower pre-load.
- Reduced blood pressure.

Cautions

Patients with suspected posterior myocardial infarction or right-ventricular infarction.

Glyceryl Trinitrate (GTN)

Contra-Indications

Hypotension (systolic blood pressure < 90mmHg in angina/myocardial infarction, or < 110 mmHg in acute heart failure).

Hypovolaemia.

Head trauma.

Cerebral haemorrhage.

Sildenafil (Viagra) and other related drugs – glyceryl trinitrate must not be given to patients who have taken sildenafil or related drugs within the previous 24 hours. Profound hypotension may occur.

Unconscious patients.

Known severe aortic or mitral stenosis.

Side Effects

Headache.

Dizziness.

Hypotension.

Additional Information

GTN tablets must be discarded 8 weeks after first opening.

NB To reduce the risk of cross contamination between patients, the nozzle of the spray must not come into contact with the patient's mouth. Wipe after each use with a detergent wipe.

*see Medicines: Best Practice checklist   **MEDS**

Glyceryl Trinitrate (GTN)   **GTN**

Dosage and Administration

The oral mucosa must be moist for GTN absorption, moisten if necessary.

Route: Sublingual tablet/spray (administer under the patient's tongue and close mouth).

ANGINA or MYOCARDIAL INFARCTION (systolic BP > 90 mmHg)

AGE	INITIAL DOSE	REPEAT DOSE	DOSE INTERVAL	VOLUME	MAXIMUM DOSE
Adult ≥18 years 400 micrograms per dose spray	400–800 micrograms	400–800 micrograms	5–10 minutes	1–2 sprays	No limit
Adult ≥18 years 300 micrograms per tablet	300 micrograms	300 micrograms	5–10 minutes	1 tablet	No limit
Adult ≥18 years 500 micrograms per tablet	500 micrograms	500 micrograms	5–10 minutes	1 tablet	No limit
Adult ≥18 years 600 micrograms per tablet	600 micrograms	600 micrograms	5–10 minutes	1 tablet	No limit

NB The effect of the first dose should be assessed over 5 minutes; further doses can be administered provided the systolic blood pressure is **>90 mmHg**. Remove the tablet if side effects occur, for example, hypotension.

Glyceryl Trinitrate (GTN)   GTN

ACUTE HEART FAILURE (systolic BP > 110 mmHg)

Route: Sublingual tablet/spray (administer under the patient's tongue and close mouth).

AGE	INITIAL DOSE	REPEAT DOSE	DOSE INTERVAL	VOLUME	MAXIMUM DOSE
Adult ≥18 years 400 micrograms per dose spray	400–800 micrograms	400–800 micrograms	5–10 minutes	1–2 sprays	6 sprays (2.4 milligrams)
Adult ≥18 years 300 micrograms per tablet	300 micrograms	300 micrograms	5–10 minutes	1 tablet	6 tablets (1.8 milligrams)
Adult ≥18 years 500 micrograms per tablet	500 micrograms	500 micrograms	5–10 minutes	1 tablet	3 tablets (1.5 milligrams)
Adult ≥18 years 600 micrograms per tablet	600 micrograms	600 micrograms	5–10 minutes	1 tablet	3 tablets (1.8 milligrams)

NB The effect of the first dose should be assessed over 5 minutes; further doses can be administered provided the systolic blood pressure is **>110 mmHg**. Remove the tablet if side effects occur, for example, hypotension.

*see Medicines: Best Practice checklist **MEDS**

Heparin (Unfractionated) **HEP**

Presentation

An ampoule of unfractionated heparin containing 5,000 units per ml.

Indications

ST-elevation myocardial infarction (STEMI) where heparin is required as adjunctive therapy with tenecteplase to reduce the risk of re-infarction.

It is extremely important that the initial bolus dose is given at the earliest opportunity prior to administration of thrombolytic agents and a heparin infusion is commenced immediately on arrival at hospital.

A further intravenous bolus dose of 1,000 units heparin may be required if a heparin infusion **HAS NOT** commenced within 45 minutes of the original bolus of thrombolytic agent.

Actions

Anticoagulant.

Contra-Indications

- **Haemophilia and other haemorrhagic disorders.**
- Thrombocytopenia.
- Recent cerebral haemorrhage.
- Severe hypertension.
- Severe liver disease.
- Oesophageal varices.
- Peptic ulcer.

Heparin (Unfractionated)   HEP

- Major trauma.
- Recent surgery to eye or nervous system.
- Acute bacterial endocarditis.
- Spinal or epidural anaesthesia.

Side Effects

Haemorrhage – major or minor.

Additional Information

Analysis of MINAP data suggests inadequate anticoagulation following pre-hospital thrombolytic treatment is associated with increased risks of re-infarction.

AT HOSPITAL it is essential that the care of the patient is handed over as soon as possible to a member of hospital staff qualified to administer the second bolus (if not already given) and commence a heparin infusion.

see Medicines: Best Practice checklist **MEDS**

Heparin (Unfractionated)   **HEP**

Dosage and Administration

Heparin dosage when administered with **TENECTEPLASE**.

Route: Intravenous single bolus unfractionated heparin.

AGE	WEIGHT	INITIAL DOSE	REPEAT DOSE	DOSE INTERVAL	VOLUME	MAXIMUM DOSE
≥18 5,000 units/ml	<67 kg	4,000 units	***See footnote**	N/A	0.8 ml	4,000 units
≥18 5,000 units/ml	≥67 kg	5,000 units	***See footnote**	N/A	1 ml	5,000 units

*A further intravenous bolus dose of 1,000 units heparin may be required if a heparin infusion **HAS NOT** commenced within 45 minutes of the original bolus of thrombolytic agent.

Hydrocortisone HYC

Presentation

Solution for injection: Hydrocortisone sodium phosphate 100mg/1ml solution for injection ampoules.

Powder for solution for injection: Hydrocortisone (as Hydrocortisone sodium succinate) 100 mg powder for reconstitution with up to 2 ml of water.

An ampoule containing 100 milligrams hydrocortisone sodium succinate for reconstitution with up to 2 ml of water.

Indications

Severe or life-threatening asthma.

Anaphylaxis.

Adrenal crisis (including Addisonian crisis) — which is a time-critical medical emergency with an associated mortality.

Adrenal crisis may occur in patients on long-term steroid therapy, either:

- as replacement therapy for adrenal insufficiency from any cause
- in long-term therapy at doses of 5+mg prednisolone, e.g. for immune-suppression.

Administer hydrocortisone to:

1. Patients in an established adrenal crisis (IV administration preferable). Ensure parenteral hydrocortisone is given prior to transportation.

see Medicines: Best Practice checklist **MEDS**

Hydrocortisone   HYC

2   Patients with suspected adrenal insufficiency or on long-term steroid therapy who have become unwell, to prevent them having an adrenal crisis. (IM administration is usually sufficient).

3   If in doubt about adrenal insufficiency, it is better to administer hydrocortisone.

Actions

Glucocorticoid drug that restores blood pressure, blood sugar, cardiac synchronicity and volume. High levels are important to survive shock. Therapeutic actions include suppression of inflammation and immune response.

Contra-Indications

Known allergy to the product/excipients.

Where a patient has adrenal crisis it is preferable to give whatever preparation is available.

Cautions

None relevant to a single dose.

Avoid intramuscular administration if patient likely to require thrombolysis.

Side Effects

Both sodium phosphate and sodium succinate solutions contain significant amounts of phosphate preservative and may cause stinging or burning sensations.

Hydrocortisone   HYC

Dosage and Administration

1. **Severe or life-threatening asthma and adrenal crisis.** NB If there is any doubt about previous steroid administration, it is better to administer further hydrocortisone. There is no toxic dose for hydrocortisone, but advanced hypocortisolaemia may rapidly prove fatal.

Route: Preferably, intravenous (**SLOW** injection over a minimum of 2 minutes to avoid side effects).

Otherwise: intramuscular (upper arm or thigh) where IV access is not possible.

Note that patients with a larger BMI will need a longer IM needle.

AGE	INITIAL DOSE	REPEAT DOSE	DOSE INTERVAL	VOLUME	MAXIMUM DOSE
Adult 100 milligrams in 1 ml	100 milligrams	NONE	N/A	1 ml	100 milligrams

Route: Intravenous (**SLOW** injection over a minimum of 2 minutes to avoid side effects)/intraosseous OR intramuscular (when IV access is impossible).

AGE	INITIAL DOSE	REPEAT DOSE	DOSE INTERVAL	VOLUME	MAXIMUM DOSE
Adult 100 milligrams in 2 ml	100 milligrams	NONE	N/A	2 ml	100 milligrams

*see Medicines: Best Practice checklist **MEDS**

Hydrocortisone   **HYC**

2. **Anaphylaxis**

Route: Intravenous (**SLOW** injection over a minimum of 2 minutes to avoid side effects)/intraosseous OR intramuscular (when IV access is impossible).

AGE	INITIAL DOSE	REPEAT DOSE	DOSE INTERVAL	VOLUME	MAXIMUM DOSE
Adult 100 milligrams in 1 ml	200 milligrams	NONE	N/A	2 ml	200 milligrams

Route: Intravenous (**SLOW** injection over a minimum of 2 minutes to avoid side effects)/intraosseous OR intramuscular (when IV access is impossible).

AGE	INITIAL DOSE	REPEAT DOSE	DOSE INTERVAL	VOLUME	MAXIMUM DOSE
Adult 100 milligrams in 2 ml	200 milligrams	NONE	N/A	4 ml	200 milligrams

Ibuprofen   IBP

Presentation

Solution or suspension containing ibuprofen 100 milligrams in 5 ml (ibuprofen 20mg in 1ml).

Tablet containing 200 milligrams or 400 milligrams ibuprofen.

Indications

Relief of mild to moderate pain.

Pyrexia with discomfort (may help to relieve the misery and often unpleasant symptoms that often accompany febrile illness, e.g. aches and pains).

Soft tissue injuries.

Best when used as part of a balanced analgesic regimen.

Actions

Analgesic (relieves pain).

Antipyretic (reduces temperature).

Anti-inflammatory (reduces inflammation).

Contra-Indications

Do **NOT** administer if the patient is:
- Dehydrated.
- Hypovolaemic.
- Known to have renal insufficiency.

*see Medicines: Best Practice checklist **MEDS**

Ibuprofen   IBP

- Patients with active upper gastrointestinal disturbance (e.g. oesophagitis, peptic ulcer, dyspepsia).
- A woman in the last trimester of pregnancy.
- A child with chickenpox.
- A patient who has previously shown hypersensitivity reactions (e.g. asthma, rhinitis, angioedema or urticaria), in response to ibuprofen, aspirin or other non-steroidal anti-inflammatory drugs.
- A patient with active peptic ulcer/haemorrhage.
- Patient with severe heart failure (NYHA Class IV), renal failure or hepatic failure.

Avoid giving further non-steroidal anti-inflammatory drugs (NSAIDs) (i.e. ibuprofen), if an NSAID containing product (e.g. diclofenac, naproxen) has been used within the previous 4 hours or if the maximum cumulative daily dose has already been given.

Do **NOT** offer non-steroidal anti-inflammatory drugs (NSAIDs) to frail or older adults with fractures.

Cautions

Asthma: Use cautiously in asthmatic patients due to the possible risk of hypersensitivity and bronchoconstriction. If an asthmatic has not used NSAIDs previously, do not use acutely in the pre-hospital setting.

Older people: Exercise caution in older patients (>65 years old) that have not used and tolerated NSAIDs recently.

- Patients with coagulation defects.
- Crohn's disease and ulcerative colitis as condition may be exacerbated.

Ibuprofen   IBP

- Avoid in patients with established ischaemic heart disease, peripheral arterial disease, cerebrovascular disease, congestive heart failure.
- Hypertension.

Side Effects
May cause nausea, vomiting and tinnitus.

Dosage and Administration
Route: Oral.

AGE	INITIAL DOSE	REPEAT DOSE	DOSE INTERVAL	VOLUME	MAXIMUM DOSE
12 years – Adult	400 milligrams	400 milligrams	8 hours	Varies	1.2 grams per 24 hours

NB

- Given up to 3 times a day, preferably following food.

see Medicines: Best Practice checklist **MEDS**

Ipratropium Bromide IPR

Presentation

Nebuliser liquid Ipratropium bromide 250 microgram per 1 ml liquid unit dose vial.

Nebuliser liquid Ipratropium bromide 500 microgram per 2 ml liquid unit dose vial (Ipratropium bromide 250 micorgram per 1 ml).

Indications

Acute severe or life-threatening asthma.

Acute asthma unresponsive to salbutamol.

Exacerbation of chronic obstructive pulmonary disease (COPD), unresponsive to salbutamol.

Actions

1. Ipratropium bromide is an antimuscarinic bronchodilator drug. It may provide short-term relief in acute asthma, but beta2 agonists (such as salbutamol) generally work more quickly.
2. Ipratropium is considered of greater benefit in:
   a. children suffering acute asthma
   b. adults suffering with COPD.

Contra-Indications

None in the emergency situation.

Cautions

Ipratropium should be used with care in patients with:
- Glaucoma (protect the eyes from mist).

Ipratropium Bromide   IPR

- Pregnancy and breastfeeding.
- Prostatic hyperplasia.

If COPD is a possibility limit nebulisation with oxygen to 6 minutes.

Side Effects

Nausea.

Dry mouth (common).

Tachycardia/arrhythmia.

Paroxysmal tightness of the chest.

Allergic reaction.

Dosage and Administration

- **In life-threatening or acute severe asthma:** undertake a **TIME CRITICAL** transfer to the **NEAREST SUITABLE RECEIVING HOSPITAL** and provide nebulisation en-route.
- If COPD is a possibility limit nebulisation to 6 minutes.

*see Medicines: Best Practice checklist **MEDS**

Ipratropium Bromide   IPR

Route: Nebuliser with 6–8 litres per minute oxygen (**refer to Oxygen**).

AGE	INITIAL DOSE	REPEAT DOSE	DOSE INTERVAL	VOLUME	MAXIMUM DOSE
Adult 250 micrograms in 1 ml	500 micrograms	NONE	N/A	2 ml	500 micrograms

Route: Nebuliser with 6–8 litres per minute oxygen (**refer to Oxygen**).

AGE	INITIAL DOSE	REPEAT DOSE	DOSE INTERVAL	VOLUME	MAXIMUM DOSE
Adult 500 micrograms in 2 ml	500 micrograms	NONE	N/A	2 ml	500 micrograms

Metoclopramide Hydrochloride   MTC

Presentation
Metoclopramide 10 milligrams/2 ml solution for injection ampoules (metoclopramide hydrochloride 5 mg per 1 ml).

Indications
The treatment of nausea or vomiting in adults aged 18 and over.

Prevention and treatment of nausea and vomiting following administration of morphine sulfate.

Actions
An anti-emetic which acts centrally as well as on the gastrointestinal tract.

Contra-Indications
- Age less than 18 years.
- Renal failure.
- Phaeochromocytoma.
- Gastrointestinal obstruction.
- Perforation/haemorrhage/3–4 days after GI surgery.
- Cases of drug overdose.

Cautions
If patient is likely to require thrombolysis then intramuscular administration of any drug should be avoided.

*see Medicines: Best Practice checklist **MEDS**

Metoclopramide Hydrochloride   MTC

Side Effects

Severe extra-pyramidal effects are more common in children and young adults.

- Drowsiness and restlessness.
- Cardiac conduction abnormalities following IV administration.
- Diarrhoea.
- Rash.

Additional Information

Metoclopramide should always be given in a separate syringe to morphine sulfate. The drugs must not be mixed.

Dosage and Administration

Route: administer by intramuscular injection or slow intravenous injection over at least 3 minutes.

AGE	INITIAL DOSE	REPEAT DOSE	DOSE INTERVAL	VOLUME	MAXIMUM DOSE
≥18 years 10 milligrams in 2 ml	10 milligrams	NONE	N/A	2 ml	10 milligrams

NB Monitor pulse, blood pressure, respiratory rate and cardiac rhythm before, during and after administration.

Midazolam   MDZ

Presentation
Midazolam oromucosal solution, 5 mg/ml, (pre-filled syringes containing 2.5 mg, 5 mg, 7.5 mg or 10 mg).

Indications
- Patients who have prolonged convulsions (lasting 5 minutes or more), OR repeated convulsions (three or more in an hour), and are **CURRENTLY CONVULSING** – not secondary to an uncorrected hypoxic or hypoglycaemic episode.
- Convulsion continuing 10 minutes after first dose of medication.

A PGD is required to administer midazolam unless a patient has their own prescribed supply. If the midazolam is prescribed for the patient the clinician MUST follow the prescriber's instructions for its administration. If a PGD is being used the document will state the clinical situation in which the medicine can be administered.

Actions
Short-acting benzodiazepine with anxiolytic, sedative and anticonvulsant properties. Onset of action is dependent on the route of administration. The buccal route onset of action is usually within 5 minutes. The sedative effect decreases from 15 minutes onwards.

*see Medicines: Best Practice checklist **MEDS**

Midazolam   MDZ

Cautions

Always check the dose of the midazolam presentation carefully.
Administration can lead to respiratory depression leading to respiratory
arrest. Susceptible patients are children, adults over 60 years and those
with chronic illness (renal, hepatic or cardiac).

Enhanced side effects when alcohol or other sedative drugs are present.

Contra-Indications

None.

Side Effects

- Respiratory depression.
- Hypotension.
- Reduced level of consciousness leading to impaired airway control.
- Confusion leading to increased agitation.
- Amnesia in some patients.

Additional Information

When administered for convulsions in known epileptic patients ask/look
to see if the patient has an individualised treatment plan or an Epilepsy
Passport. Aim to follow patient's own treatment plan when possible and
effective.

Carefully monitor vital signs for delayed respiratory or cardiovascular
side effects as the effect of the midazolam and other drugs such as
rectal diazepam reach a peak effect.

Midazolam

MDZ

Dosage and Administration
Convulsions

Route: Buccal.

AGE	INITIAL DOSE	REPEAT DOSE	DOSE INTERVAL	VOLUME	MAX DOSE
Adult 5 milligrams in 1 ml	10 milligrams	10 milligrams	10 mins	2 ml pre-filled syringe	20 milligrams

*see Medicines: Best Practice checklist **MEDS**

Misoprostol   **MIS**

Presentation

Tablet containing misoprostol:

- 200 micrograms.

Indications

- Post-partum haemorrhage (PPH) within 24 hours of birth where bleeding from the uterus is uncontrollable by uterine massage and use of Syntometrine.
- Life-threatening obstetric bleeding less than 24 weeks pregnant where a miscarriage has been **confirmed** (e.g. confirmed by ultrasound scan, or when a miscarriage is being managed at home with medical treatment or a fetus has definitely been passed and seen). Life-threatening bleeding is normally more than 500mls **OR** when signs of shock are present.

NB Misoprostol should only be used if other oxytocics are unavailable or if they have been ineffective at reducing haemorrhage after 15 minutes.

NB Misoprostol should be used as first-line drug treatment for PPH in pre-eclampsia or hypertension where BP is 140/90 mmHg or more (or where systolic BP alone is 150 mmHg or more). Syntometrine (ergometrine and oxytocin) is contra-indicated in hypertension.

Actions

Stimulates contraction of the uterus.

Onset of action 7–10 minutes.

Misoprostol

Contra-indications
- Any bleeding in pregnancy if there is any suspicion that the fetus or embryo is in the uterus ('in utero').
- In labour, prior to the birth of the baby (with a multiple pregnancy, ensure all babies have delivered).
- Known hypersensitivity to misoprostol.
- Secondary post-partum haemorrhage (excess bleeding more than 24 hours after delivery of the baby).

Side Effects
- Abdominal pain.
- Nausea and vomiting.
- Diarrhoea.
- Pyrexia.
- Shivering.

Additional Information
Oxytocin and misoprostol reduce bleeding from a pregnant uterus through different pathways; therefore, if one drug has not been effective after 15 minutes, the other may be administered in addition.

*see Medicines: Best Practice checklist   **MEDS**

Misoprostol   **MIS**

Dosage and Administration

- Administer sublingually unless the patient is unable to maintain their airway.

- The vaginal route is not appropriate in post-partum haemorrhage or for miscarriage, but the rectal route may be considered when appropriate (e.g. impaired consciousness).

Route: Sublingual.

AGE	INITIAL DOSE	REPEAT DOSE	DOSE INTERVAL	VOLUME	MAX DOSE
Adult 200 micrograms per tablet	800 micrograms	**None**	N/A	4 tablets	800 micrograms

Route: Rectal.

> **NB** At the time of publication there is no rectal preparation of misoprostol – therefore the same tablets can be administered sublingually or rectally.

AGE	INITIAL DOSE	REPEAT DOSE	DOSE INTERVAL	VOLUME	MAX DOSE
Adult 200 micrograms per tablet	800 micrograms	**None**	N/A	4 tablets	800 micrograms

Morphine Sulfate   MOR

Presentation
Solution for injection ampoules: morphine sulfate 10 mg/ml (morphine sulfate 10 mg per 1 ml).

Oral solution: morphine sulfate 10 mg/5 ml (morphine sulfate 2 mg per 1 ml).

Indications
- Pain associated with suspected myocardial infarction (analgesic of first choice).
- Severe pain as a component of a balanced analgesia regimen.

The decision about which analgesia and which route should be guided by clinical judgement. Refer to **Pain Management in Adults** and **Pain Management in Children**.

Indications Specific to Adults at the End of Life
Using ambulance service issue morphine for end of life should only be followed in situations where:

- A patient's own medication for pain or breathlessness has not been prescribed.
- The patient's own medication is not yet available or has run out.
- Medicines are in place without a patient-specific document signed by an independent prescriber.

Wherever possible, liaison should occur with palliative care/nursing teams in line with local pathways, particularly if 'anticipatory' or 'just in case' medicines are prescribed and are available.

see Medicines: Best Practice checklist **MEDS**

Morphine Sulfate MOR

Consider discussing with a senior clinician for advice and support, preferably a clinician with expertise in end of life care, before administering morphine. Follow local pathways to access senior clinician support.

If a patient has their own prescribed morphine, use this.

For both breathlessness and pain management in adults, refer to the **End of Life Care** guideline.

Breathlessness

● Patient is at end of life, and is distressed and breathless.

Reversible causes of breathlessness should always be considered first.

If you are unable to access rapid community/palliative care, morphine should be administered.

Pain

● Patient is at end of life and is in pain.

Actions

Morphine is a strong opioid analgesic.

Morphine produces sedation, euphoria and analgesia; it may both depress respiration and induce hypotension.

Histamine is released following morphine administration and this may contribute to its vasodilatory effects. This may also account for the urticaria and bronchoconstriction that are sometimes seen.

Actions Specific to Adults at the End of Life

Morphine is particularly useful for treating continuous, severe musculoskeletal and soft tissue pain, and for distress associated with breathlessness at end of life.

Morphine Sulfate — MOR

Contra-Indications

Do **NOT** administer morphine in the following circumstances:

- Children under 1 year of age.
- Respiratory depression (adult <10 breaths per minute, child <20 breaths per minute).
- Hypotension (actual, not estimated, systolic blood pressure <90 mmHg in adults, <80 mmHg in school children, <70 mmHg in pre-school children).
- Head injury with significantly impaired level of consciousness (e.g. below P on the AVPU scale or below 9 on the GCS).
- Known hypersensitivity to morphine.

Contra-Indications Specific to Adults at the End of Life

Once the clinician has confirmed the patient has pain and/or breathlessness, and is at the end of life, then the benefits of morphine clearly outweigh treatment-related adverse effects. Cautions and contra-indications do not generally apply; the focus should be on symptom control for the patient to ensure a peaceful and dignified death. It is important that palliative care specialists involved in the patient's care should be consulted as part of the assessment process. The use of the subcutaneous route also reduces the likelihood of some of these adverse effects.

Cautions

Known severe renal or hepatic impairment — smaller doses may be used carefully and titrated to effect.

see Medicines: Best Practice checklist **MEDS**

Morphine Sulfate   MOR

Use with **extreme** caution (minimal doses) during pregnancy. **NB** Not to be used for labour pain where Nitrous Oxide (Entonox®) is the analgesic of choice.

Use morphine **WITH GREAT CAUTION** in patients with chest injuries, particularly those with any respiratory difficulty, although if respiration is inhibited by pain, analgesia may actually improve respiratory status.

Any patients with other respiratory problems (e.g. asthma, COPD).

Head injury. Agitation following head injury may be due to acute brain injury, hypoxia or pain. The decision to administer analgesia to an agitated head injured patient is a clinical one. It is vital that if such a patient receives opioids they are closely monitored since opioids can cause disproportionate respiratory depression, which may ultimately lead to an elevated intracranial pressure through a raised arterial pCO_2.

Acute alcohol intoxication. All opioid drugs potentiate the central nervous system depressant effects of alcohol and they should therefore be used with great caution in patients who have consumed significant quantities of alcohol.

Medications. Prescribed antidepressants, sedatives or major tranquillisers may potentiate the respiratory and cardiovascular depressant effects of morphine.

Morphine may not be the appropriate treatment for a headache when the cause for the headache is uncertain, for example, a possible migraine.

Smaller doses should be considered for patients weighing less than 50kg, and for frail and/or older patients who may be more susceptible to complications.

Morphine Sulfate — MOR

Cautions Specific to Adults at the End of Life

For pain in the last days or hours of life when the patient is in the dying phase, morphine may be given with caution for patients with a systolic blood pressure of 90mmHg or less.

If the patient has been prescribed their own 'anticipatory' or 'just in case' medications for pain, and this medicine is available, then administer the medication from the patient's own supply, in liaison with the palliative care or nursing team.

Check for prior opioid use before administration to avoid overdosing the patient.

Side Effects

- Respiratory depression.
- Cardiovascular depression.
- Nausea and vomiting.
- Drowsiness.
- Pupillary constriction.

Additional Information

Morphine injection is a Class A controlled drug under Schedule 2 of the Misuse of Drugs Regulations 2001. It is subject to the Safe Custody Regulations 1973, and must be stored securely with its movements recorded in a controlled drug register. Its administration and supply is strictly controlled, and it may only be possessed and administered by healthcare professionals authorised in the legislation.

Unused morphine in open vials or syringes must be discarded in the presence of a witness.

*see Medicines: Best Practice checklist **MEDS**

Morphine Sulfate   **MOR**

Morphine is not licensed for use in children but its use has been approved by the Medicines and Healthcare Products Regulatory Agency (MHRA) for 'off label' use. This means that it can legally be administered under these guidelines by paramedics.

Additional Information Specific to Adults at the End of Life

Consider, identify and treat any reversible causes of pain and/or breathlessness.

Special Precautions

Naloxone can be used to reverse morphine related respiratory or cardiovascular depression. It should be carefully titrated after assessment and appropriate management of ABC for that particular patient and situation, refer to **Naloxone Hydrochloride**.

Morphine frequently induces nausea or vomiting which may be potentiated by the movement of the ambulance. Titrating to the lowest dose to achieve analgesia will reduce the risk of vomiting. The use of an anti-emetic should also be considered whenever administering any opioid analgesic, refer to **Ondansetron** and **Metoclopramide Hydrochloride**.

Special Precautions specific to Adults at the End of Life

The use of Naloxone in palliative care is not routinely practised and is only indicated in circumstances where a clinician suspects opioid induced toxicity, from intentional or unintentional overdose. The aim is to reverse life-threatening respiratory depression only i.e. if the

Morphine Sulfate MOR

respiratory rate is <8 breaths per minute and the patient is unconscious and or cyanosed.

Refer to the **End of Life Care** guideline opioid administration in the last hours of life and for death after drug administration.

Dosage and Administration

Administration must be in conjunction with pain score monitoring, refer to **Pain Management in Adults** and **Pain Management in Children**.

Intravenous morphine takes a minimum of 2–3 minutes before starting to take effect, reaching its peak between 10 and 20 minutes.

The absorption of intramuscular, subcutaneous or oral morphine is variable, particularly in patients with major trauma, shock and cardiac conditions; these routes should preferably be avoided if the circumstances favour intravenous or intraosseous administration.

Morphine **should be** diluted with sodium chloride 0.9% to make a concentration of 10 milligrams in 10 ml (1 milligram in 1 ml) unless it is being administered by the intramuscular or subcutaneous route when it should not be diluted.

ADULTS – If pain is not reduced to a tolerable level after 10 milligrams of IV/IO morphine, then further **2 milligram** doses may be administered by slow IV/IO injection every 5 minutes to **20 milligrams maximum**. The patient should be closely observed throughout the remaining treatment and transfer. Smaller doses should be considered for lightweight children over age 12 and for older, frail patients who may be more susceptible to complications.

CHILDREN – The doses and volumes given below are for the initial and maximum doses. Administer **0.1 ml/kg** (equal to **100 micrograms/kg**) as

see Medicines: Best Practice checklist **MEDS**

Morphine Sulfate   MOR

an initial slow IV injection over 2 minutes. If pain is not reduced to a tolerable level after 5 minutes then a further dose of up to **100 micrograms/kg**, titrated to response, may be repeated (**maximum dose 200 micrograms/kg**).

NOTE: Peak effect of each dose may not occur until 10–20 minutes after administration.

Intravenous/intraosseous (**NOT** end of life)

Route: Intravenous/intraosseous – administer by slow IV injection (rate of approximately 2 milligrams per minute up to appropriate dose for age). Observe the patient for at least 5 minutes after completion of initial dose before repeating the dose if required.

Smaller initial doses (e.g. 1 milligram) should be used for frail and/or older patients.

AGE	INITIAL DOSE	REPEAT DOSE	DOSE INTERVAL	DILUTED CONCENTRATION	VOLUME	MAX DOSE
Adult ≥ 50kg	10 milligrams	10 milligrams	5 minutes	10 milligrams in 10 ml	10 ml	20 milligrams
Adult < 50kg	2 milligrams	2 milligrams	4 minutes	10 milligrams in 10 ml	2 ml	10 milligrams

Subcutaneous/intramuscular (**NOT** end of life)

Route: Subcutaneous/intramuscular.

NB For patients with major trauma, shock, or cardiac conditions, administer via IV/IO routes. Only administer via the subcutaneous or intramuscular route if the IV/IO routes are not accessible.

Morphine Sulfate — MOR

For administration by the subcutaneous or intramuscular route, do not dilute the morphine, as more than 1 ml of fluid injected into the site of administration is not recommended. The effects of SC/IM morphine are evident after 15–20 minutes.

Smaller initial doses (e.g. 1 milligram) should be used for frail and/or older patients.

AGE	INITIAL DOSE	REPEAT DOSE	DOSE INTERVAL	UNDILUTED CONCENTRATION	VOLUME	MAX DOSE
Adult ≥ 50kg	10 milligrams	10 milligrams	60 minutes	10 milligrams in 1 ml	1 ml	20 milligrams
Adult < 50kg	5 milligrams	5 milligrams	60 minutes	10 milligrams in 1 ml	0.5 ml	10 milligrams

Oral (NOT end of life)

Route: Oral.

NB Only administer via the oral route in patients with major trauma, shock or cardiac conditions if the IV/IO routes are not accessible.

AGE	INITIAL DOSE	REPEAT DOSE	DOSE INTERVAL	CONCENTRATION	VOLUME	MAX DOSE
Adult ≥ 12 years	20 milligrams	20 milligrams	60 minutes	10 milligrams in 5 ml	10 ml	40 milligrams

*see Medicines: Best Practice checklist **MEDS**

Morphine Sulfate   **MOR**

Pain End of Life – Subcutaneous/intramuscular

Route: Subcutaneous/intramuscular.

The subcutaneous route is the preferred route for pain management at the end of life. However, the intramuscular route can also be used.

For administration by the subcutaneous or intramuscular route, do not dilute the morphine, as more than 1 ml of fluid injected into the site of administration is not recommended. The effects of SC/IM morphine are evident after 15–20 minutes.

AGE	INITIAL DOSE	REPEAT DOSE	DOSE INTERVAL	CONCEN-TRATION	VOLUME	MAX DOSE
Adult ≥18 years For adults with pre-scriptions available	Administer prescribed dose. If dose range given, administer lowest dose or in line with previous dose	Seek senior clinical advice	N/A	N/A	N/A	N/A
Adult ≥18 years For opioid naive patients or those with an unknown opioid tolerance	2.5 milligrams	Seek senior clinical advice	N/A	N/A	N/A	N/A
Adult ≥18 years For opioid naive/ patients with an unknown opioid tolerance who also have severe respi-ratory compromise	1 milligram	Seek senior clinical advice	N/A	N/A	N/A	N/A

Morphine Sulfate — MOR

AGE	INITIAL DOSE	REPEAT DOSE	DOSE INTERVAL	CONCENTRATION	VOLUME	MAX DOSE
Adult ≥18 years For patients who are on a known dose of a strong regular opioid. If the patient is already on opioids, then treatment for breakthrough pain is 1/6 of the total 24 hour dosage. Refer to Patient Specific Direction/ Just In Case	2.5 milligrams – 5 milligrams	Seek senior clinical advice	N/A	N/A	N/A	N/A

Pain End of Life – Oral
Route: Oral.

AGE	INITIAL DOSE	REPEAT DOSE	DOSE INTERVAL	CONCENTRATION	VOLUME	MAX DOSE
Adult ≥18 years For adults with prescriptions available	Administer prescribed dose. If dose range given, administer lowest dose or in line with previous dose	Seek senior clinical advice	N/A	N/A	N/A	N/A

*see Medicines: Best Practice checklist **MEDS**

Morphine Sulfate   MOR

AGE	INITIAL DOSE	REPEAT DOSE	DOSE INTERVAL	CONCEN-TRATION	VOLUME	MAX DOSE
Adult ≥18 years For opioid naive patients or those with an unknown opioid tolerance	5 milligrams in 2.5 millilitres	Seek senior clinical advice	N/A	N/A	N/A	N/A
Adult ≥18 years For opioid naive/ patients with an unknown opioid tolerance who also have severe respiratory compromise	2.5 milligrams in 1.25 millilitres	Seek senior clinical advice	N/A	N/A	N/A	N/A
Adult ≥18 years For patients who are on a known dose of a strong regular opioid	Administer the usual breakthrough dose or 1/6 of the total 24 hour dosage of oral morphine	Seek senior clinical advice	N/A	N/A	N/A	N/A

Breathlessness End of Life – Subcutaneous/intramuscular

Route: Subcutaneous/intramuscular.

Reversible causes of breathlessness should always be considered first.

Consider discussing with a senior clinician for advice and support, preferably a clinician with expertise in end of life care before

Morphine Sulfate MOR

administering morphine for breathlessness. Follow local pathways to access senior clinician support.

Patient at end of life, in distress, and breathless.
Patient has no anticipatory medicines in place.
You are unable to access rapid community/palliative care.

AGE	INITIAL DOSE	REPEAT DOSE	DOSE INTERVAL	CONCEN-TRATION	VOLUME	MAX DOSE
Adult ≥18 years	1 milligram to 2.5 milligrams	Seek senior clinical advice	N/A	N/A	N/A	N/A

If the patient remains breathless, consider prompt referral to community/palliative care to consider administration of appropriate medications such as subcutaneous morphine administration via a syringe driver. Follow local procedures for access to local pathways and how to access senior clinician support. Other medications may need to be administered for breathlessness and anxiety such as lorazepam, midazolam, antiemetic-haloperidol and a stimulant laxative (senna).

Breathlessness End of Life – Oral
Route: Oral
Reversible causes of breathlessness should always be considered first.

Consider discussing with a senior clinician for advice and support, preferably a clinician with expertise in end of life care before administering morphine for breathlessness. Follow local pathways to access senior clinician support.

*see Medicines: Best Practice checklist   **MEDS**

Morphine Sulfate   **MOR**

Patient at end of life, in distress, and breathless.

Patient has no anticipatory medicines in place.

You are unable to access rapid community/palliative care.

NB Lower doses should be considered for patients ‹50kg or opioid naïve.

AGE	INITIAL DOSE	REPEAT DOSE	DOSE INTERVAL	CONCEN-TRATION	VOLUME	MAX DOSE
Adults who are opioid naive (not currently taking opioids)	Morphine sulfate oral solution immediate release 2.5 milligrams to 5 milligrams	Seek senior clinical advice	N/A	N/A	N/A	N/A
Adults already taking regular opioids for other reasons	Morphine sulfate oral solution 5 milligrams to 10 milligrams	Seek senior clinical advice	N/A	N/A	N/A	N/A

If the patient remains breathless, consider prompt referral to community/palliative care to consider administration of appropriate medications such as subcutaneous morphine administration via a syringe driver. Follow local procedures for access to local pathways and how to access senior clinician support. Other medications may need to be administered for breathlessness and anxiety such as lorazepam, midazolam, antiemetic-haloperidol and a stimulant laxative (senna).

Naloxone Hydrochloride — NLX

Presentation
Naloxone hydrochloride 400 micrograms per 1 ml ampoule.

Indications

The reversal of acute opioid or opiate toxicity for respiratory arrest or respiratory depression.

Unconsciousness, associated with respiratory depression of unknown cause, where opioid overdose is a possibility. Refer to **Altered Level of Consciousness**.

In cardiac arrest, where opioid toxicity is considered to be the likely cause.

Patients exposed to high-potency veterinary or anaesthetic preparations should be given naloxone urgently if:

- Consciousness is impaired

OR

- Exposure occurred within the last 10 minutes, even if asymptomatic.

If an antidote is supplied with the opioid medication, such as diprenorphine (Revivon) or naloxone, it should be administered immediately.

Actions
Complete or partial reversal of the respiratory depression effects of opioid drugs.

*see Medicines: Best Practice checklist **MEDS**

Naloxone Hydrochloride　　NLX

The aim of naloxone administration is to restore adequate respirations but not necessarily to restore full consciousness.

Contra-indications

Neonates born to opioid addicted mothers can result in serious withdrawal effects. Emphasis should be on bag-valve-mask ventilation and oxygenation.

Side Effects

- In patients who are physically dependent on opioids, naloxone may precipitate violent withdrawal symptoms, including cardiac arrhythmias. It is better, in these cases, to titrate the dose of naloxone as described in the dosing charts in this guideline to effectively reverse the cardiac and respiratory depression, but still leave the patient in a 'groggy' state with regular reassessment of ventilation and circulation.

- Vomiting is a common side effect following naloxone administration, ensure access to suction.

Additional Information

When indicated, naloxone can be administered via the intravenous, intramuscular, intraosseous, subcutaneous or intranasal route. Very ill patients will require intravenous naloxone to ensure rapid absorption of the total dose.

Refer to local procedures/product instructions for the route of administration and for intranasal dose and time intervals.

Naloxone Hydrochloride   NLX

For intramuscular administration, the drug should be **undiluted** (into the outer aspect of the thigh or upper arm). Absorption may be unpredictable.

All cases of opioid overdose should be transported to hospital, even if the initial response to naloxone has been good. The duration of action of naloxone is usually 30 to 90 minutes and this is shorter than some opioids such as methadone; therefore additional doses of naloxone may be necessary to maintain reversal of opioid induced respiratory depression. Patients who have ingested methadone require observation for at least 8 hours following overdose to prevent accidental death. If the patient refuses to go to hospital, consider, if the patient consents, a loading dose of **800 micrograms IM** to minimise the risk described above. For patients who refuse transfer to hospital if possible leave in the care of a responsible adult and leave an advice leaflet advising of action to be taken in the event that the symptoms return.

Some patients at risk of opiate misuse (or their carers) may have been given take home naloxone as a harm-reduction measure.

The large difference in doses between adult and children reflects the likely aetiology of the opiate ingestion and aims of treatment.

In children aged under 12, the aetiology is likely to be accidental ingestion and they are unlikely to be dependent on opiates (unless they are an end of life care patient) so the aim is to totally reverse the opiate. If you feel the child needs further doses in the same episode of illness they must be reviewed by a senior healthcare professional; seek senior clinical advice.

see Medicines: Best Practice checklist **MEDS**

Naloxone Hydrochloride NLX

Adults are more likely to be dependant opiate users and may become aggressive if the opiate is reversed, so the aim is a controlled reversal.

Methadone is a long-acting synthetic opioid that is used in opioid harm reduction and substance misuse programmes. Methadone has an elimination half-life of between 15 and 60 hours, in contrast to the shorter-acting naloxone which has a half-life of 1 to 1.5 hours.

Cautions for End of Life Care Patients

The use of naloxone in palliative care is not routinely practised, as patients on regular opioids can be physically dependant. It is only indicated in circumstances where a clinician suspects opioid induced toxicity, from intentional or unintentional overdose. The aim is to reverse life-threatening respiratory depression only i.e. if the respiratory rate is <8 breaths per minute and the patient is unconscious and or cyanosed. Refer to **End of Life Care**.

Dosage and Administration: IV/IO

Respiratory arrest/respiratory depression

Route: Intravenous/intraosseous

For adults who may be opiate dependant: administer **slowly**, 1 ml at a time. Titrate to response relieving respiratory depression but maintain patient in 'groggy' state. For known or potentially aggressive adults suffering respiratory depression: dilute up to 800 micrograms (2 ml) of naloxone into 8 ml of water for injections or sodium chloride 0.9% to a total volume of 10 ml and administer **slowly**, titrating to response, 1 ml at a time.

Naloxone Hydrochloride — NLX

If there is no response after the initial dose, repeat the dose, up to the maximum dose or until an effect is noted.

NB The duration of action of naloxone is short.

PLEASE NOTE: For children using the IV/IO route, the initial dose is much higher than that for adults with the aim of totally reversing the opiate effect as quickly as possible. Please read dosages carefully.

Seek advice to exceed the maximum dose as per local procedures.

AGE	INITIAL DOSE	REPEAT DOSE	DOSE INTERVAL	VOLUME	MAX DOSE
≥12 years 400 micrograms in 1 ml	400 micrograms	400 micrograms	3 minutes	1 ml	4,000 micrograms

Cardiac arrest, where opioid toxicity is considered to be the likely cause

Route: Intravenous/intraosseous

In cardiac arrest, children or adults, repeat up to maximum dose until ROSC achieved.

AGE	INITIAL DOSE	REPEAT DOSE	DOSE INTERVAL	VOLUME	MAX DOSE
≥12 years 400 micrograms in 1 ml	400 micrograms	800 micrograms	1 minute	1 ml	10,000 micrograms

*see Medicines: Best Practice checklist **MEDS**

Naloxone Hydrochloride **NLX**

Dosage and Administration: IM

Respiratory arrest/respiratory depression where the IV/IO route is unavailable or the ambulance clinician is not trained to administer drugs via the IV/IO route.

Route: Intramuscular/subcutaneous. Only use this route if the IV/IO route is not available.

If there is no response after the initial dose, give up to the maximum dose or until an effect is noted. **NB** the half-life of naloxone is short.

For children: give the full dose with the aim of totally reversing the opiate effects.

Administering large volumes via the intramuscular route could lead to poor absorption and/or tissue damage. Therefore, divide the dose where necessary and practicable. Vary the site of injection for repeated doses.

AGE	INITIAL DOSE	REPEAT DOSE	DOSE INTERVAL	VOLUME	MAX DOSE
≥12 years 400 micrograms in 1 ml	400 micrograms	400 micrograms	3 minutes	1 ml	4,000 micrograms

Nitrous Oxide (Entonox®) NOO

Presentation

Nitrous Oxide (Entonox®) 1ml per 1ml medical gas is a combination of nitrous oxide 50% and oxygen 50%. It is stored in medical cylinders that have a blue body with white shoulders.

Indications

Moderate to severe pain.

Labour pains.

Actions

Inhaled analgesic agent.

Contra-indications

Nitrous oxide may have a deleterious effect if administered to patients with closed body cavities containing air since nitrous oxide diffuses into such a space with a resulting increase in pressure.

Do not give Entonox to patients with:

- Severe head injuries with impaired consciousness due to possible presence of intracranial air.
- Decompression sickness (the bends) where Entonox can cause nitrogen bubbles within the blood stream to expand, aggravating the problem further. Consider anyone that has been diving within the previous 24 hours to be at risk.
- Violently disturbed psychiatric patients.

169

MEDS

*see Medicines: Best Practice checklist

Nitrous Oxide (Entonox®)   NOO

- An intraocular injection of gas within the last eight weeks. Check to see if these patients have an information leaflet, card or wristband. The information leaflet may advise that Nitrous Oxide can be administered less than eight weeks after intraocular injection of gas.

- Abdominal pain where intestinal obstruction is suspected.

Cautions

Any patient at risk of having a pneumothorax, pneumomediastinum and/ or a pneumoperitoneum (e.g. polytrauma, penetrating torso injury).

Side Effects

Minimal side effects.

Additional Information

Prolonged use for more than 24 hours, or more frequently than every four days, can lead to vitamin B12 deficiency.

Administration of Entonox should be in conjunction with pain score monitoring.

Entonox's advantages include:

- Rapid analgesic effect with minimal side effects.

- No cardiorespiratory depression.

- Self-administered.

- Analgesic effect rapidly wears off.

- The 50% oxygen concentration is valuable in many medical and trauma conditions.

Nitrous Oxide (Entonox®) NOO

- Entonox can be administered whilst preparing to deliver other analgesics.

The usual precautions must be followed with regard to caring for the Entonox equipment and the cylinder MUST be inverted several times before use to mix the gases when temperatures are low.

Dosage and Administration

Adults:

- Entonox should be self-administered via a facemask or mouthpiece, after suitable instruction. It takes about **3–5 minutes** to be effective, but it may be **5–10 minutes** before maximum effect is achieved.

Children:

- Entonox is effective in children provided they are capable of following the administration instructions and can activate the demand valve.

*see Medicines: Best Practice checklist   MEDS

Ondansetron   ODT

Presentation

Ampoule containing 4 milligrams of ondansetron (as hydrochloride) in 2 ml.

Ampoule containing 8 milligrams of ondansetron (as hydrochloride) in 4 ml.

NB Both these preparations share the same concentration (2 milligrams in 1 ml).

Indications

Adults:

- Prevention and treatment of opiate-induced nausea and vomiting (e.g. morphine sulfate).
- Treatment of nausea or vomiting.

Children:

- Prevention and treatment of opiate-induced nausea and vomiting (e.g. morphine sulfate).
- For travel associated nausea or vomiting.

Actions

An anti-emetic that blocks 5HT receptors both centrally and in the gastrointestinal tract.

Contra-Indications

Known sensitivity to ondansetron.

Infants <1 month old.

Ondansetron ODT

Cautions
QT interval prolongation (avoid concomitant administration of drugs that prolong QT interval).

Hepatic impairment.

Pregnancy.

Breastfeeding.

Side Effects
- Hiccups.
- Constipation.
- Flushing.
- Hypotension.
- Chest pain.
- Arrhythmias.
- Bradycardia.
- Headache.
- Seizures.
- Movement disorders.
- Injection site reactions.

Additional Information
Ondansetron should always be given in a separate syringe to morphine sulfate – the drugs must **NOT** be mixed.

Ondansetron should **NOT** be routinely administered in the management of childhood gastroenteritis (refer to **Paediatric Gastroenteritis**).

*see Medicines: Best Practice checklist   **MEDS**

Ondansetron   ODT

Vomiting can be a symptom of a more serious problem. If a patient is sufficiently unwell that they require parenteral anti-emetics, the Paramedic must seek further advice from a specialist or a GP before making the decision to leave them on scene with Ondansetron.

Dosage and Administration

Note: Two preparations exist (4 mg in 2 ml and 8 mg in 4 ml). They share the same concentration, that is 2 milligrams in 1 ml.

Route: Intravenous (**SLOW** IV injection over 2 minutes)/intramuscular.

AGE	INITIAL DOSE	REPEAT DOSE	DOSE INTERVAL	VOLUME	MAXIMUM DOSE
≥12 years – Adult 2 milligrams in 1 ml	4 milligrams	NONE	N/A	2 ml	4 milligrams

NB Monitor pulse, blood pressure, respiratory rate and cardiac rhythm before, during and after administration.

Oxygen OXG

Presentation

Oxygen (O_2) is a gas provided in compressed form in a cylinder. It is also available in liquid form, in a system adapted for ambulance use. It is fed via a regulator and flow meter to the patient by means of plastic tubing and an oxygen mask/nasal cannulae.

Indications

Children

- Significant illness and/or injury.

Adults

- Critical illnesses requiring high levels of supplemental oxygen (refer to **High levels of supplemental oxygen for adults with critical illnesses**).
- Serious illnesses requiring moderate levels of supplemental oxygen if the patient is hypoxaemic (refer **Moderate levels of supplemental oxygen for adults with serious illnesses if the patient is hypoxaemic**).
- COPD and other conditions requiring controlled or low-dose oxygen therapy (refer to **Controlled or low-dose supplemental oxygen for adults with COPD and other conditions requiring controlled or low-dose oxygen therapy**).

*see Medicines: Best Practice checklist **MEDS**

Oxygen   OXG

- Conditions for which patients should be monitored closely but oxygen therapy is not required unless the patient is hypoxaemic (refer to **No supplemental oxygen required for adults with these conditions unless the patient is hypoxaemic but patients should be monitored closely**).

Actions

Essential for cell metabolism. Adequate tissue oxygenation is essential for normal physiological function.

Oxygen assists in reversing hypoxia, by raising the concentration of inspired oxygen. Hypoxia will, however, only improve if respiratory effort or ventilation and tissue perfusion are adequate.

If ventilation is inadequate or absent, assisting or completely taking over the patient's ventilation is essential to reverse hypoxia.

Contra-indications

Explosive environments.

Cautions

Oxygen increases the fire hazard at the scene of an incident.

Defibrillation – ensure pads firmly applied to reduce spark hazard.

Side Effects

Non-humidified O_2 is drying and irritating to mucous membranes over a period of time.

In patients with COPD there is a risk that even moderately high doses of inspired oxygen can produce increased carbon dioxide levels which may cause respiratory depression and this may lead to respiratory arrest.

Oxygen   OXG

Refer to **Controlled or low-dose supplemental oxygen for adults with COPD and other conditions requiring controlled or low-dose oxygen therapy** for guidance.

Dosage and Administration

- Measure oxygen saturation (SpO$_2$) in all patients using pulse oximetry.
- For the administration of **moderate** levels of supplemented oxygen nasal cannulae are recommended in preference to a simple face mask as they offer a more flexible dose range.
- Patients with tracheostomy or previous laryngectomy may require alternative appliances (e.g. tracheostomy masks).
- Entonox may be administered when required.
- Document oxygen administration.

Children

- **ALL** children with significant illness and/or injury should receive **HIGH** levels of supplementary oxygen.

Adults

- Administer the initial oxygen dose until a reliable oxygen saturation reading is obtained.
- If the desired oxygen saturation cannot be maintained with a simple face mask, change to a high concentration oxygen mask.
- For dosage and administration of supplemental oxygen refer to the dosage tables in this guideline.

*see Medicines: Best Practice checklist **MEDS**

Oxygen   OXG

- For conditions where **NO** supplemental oxygen is required unless the patient is hypoxaemic refer to **No supplemental oxygen required for adults with these conditions unless the patient is hypoxaemic but patients should be monitored closely**.

- BTS guidance states that a sudden reduction of more than 3% in a patient's oxygen saturation within the target saturation range should prompt fuller assessment of the patient because this may be the first evidence of an acute illness.

- Some people aged above 70 years may have saturation measurements in the range of 92–94% when clinically stable. These people do not require oxygen therapy unless the oxygen saturation falls below the level that is known to be normal for the individual patient.

Oxygen — OXG

High levels of supplemental oxygen for adults with critical illnesses

Target saturation 94–98%

Administer the initial oxygen dose until the vital signs are normal, then reduce oxygen dose and aim for target saturation within the range of 94–98% as per table below.

Condition	Initial dose	Method of administration
Cardiac arrest or resuscitation: – basic life support – advanced life support – foreign body airway obstruction – traumatic cardiac arrest – maternal resuscitation.	Maximum dose until the vital signs are normal	Bag-valve-mask
Carbon monoxide poisoning	Maximum dose – patients with carbon monoxide poisoning should receive high concentration until fully recovered and do not reduce the flow to achieve SpO$_2$ of 94–98%	High concentration oxygen mask

NOTE – Some oxygen saturation monitors cannot differentiate between carboxyhaemoglobin and oxyhaemoglobin owing to carbon monoxide poisoning

Oxygen

High levels of supplemental oxygen for adults with critical illnesses

Target saturation 94–98%

Administer the initial oxygen dose until the vital signs are normal, then reduce oxygen dose and aim for target saturation within the range of 94–98% as per table below.

Condition	Initial dose	Method of administration
● Major trauma: – abdominal trauma – burns and scalds – electrocution – head trauma – limb trauma – spinal injury and spinal cord injury – pelvic trauma – the immersion incident – thoracic trauma – trauma in pregnancy.	15 litres per minute	High concentration oxygen mask

*see Medicines: Best Practice checklist

Oxygen

High levels of supplemental oxygen for adults with critical illnesses

Target saturation 94–98%

Administer the initial oxygen dose until the vital signs are normal, then reduce oxygen dose and aim for target saturation within the range of **94–98%** as per table below.

Condition	Initial dose	Method of administration
- Anaphylaxis - Decompression illness (remain on high level oxygen until specialist advice received) - Major pulmonary haemorrhage - Sepsis (e.g. meningococcal septicaemia) - Shock - Drowning	15 litres per minute	High concentration oxygen mask
- Active convulsion - Hypothermia	Administer 15 litres per minute until a reliable SpO$_2$ measurement can be obtained and the adjust oxygen flow to aim for target saturation within the range of **94–98%**	High concentration oxygen mask

Oxygen

Moderate levels of supplemental oxygen for adults with serious illnesses if the patient is hypoxaemic

Target saturation 94–98%	Administer the initial oxygen dose until a reliable SpO$_2$ measurement is available, then adjust oxygen flow to aim for target saturation within the range of **94–98%** as per the table below.		
Condition	**Initial dose**		**Method of administration**
• Acute hypoxaemia (cause not yet diagnosed)	**SpO$_2$ <85%** 10–15 litres per minute		High concentration oxygen mask
• Deterioration of lung fibrosis or other interstitial lung disease • Acute asthma • Acute heart failure • Pneumonia • Lung cancer • Postoperative breathlessness • Pulmonary embolism	**SpO$_2$ ≥85–93%** 2–6 litres per minute		Nasal cannulae
• Pleural effusions • Pneumothorax • Severe anaemia • Sickle cell crisis	**SpO$_2$ ≥85–93%** 5–10 litres per minute		Simple face mask

*see Medicines: Best Practice checklist

OXG

Oxygen

Controlled or low-dose supplemental oxygen for adults with COPD and other conditions requiring controlled or low-dose oxygen therapy

Target saturation 88–92% — Administer the initial oxygen dose until a reliable SpO_2 measurement is available, then adjust oxygen flow to aim for target saturation within the range of **88–92%** or **pre-specified range** detailed on the patient's alert card, as per the table below.

Condition	Initial dose	Method of administration
Chronic obstructive pulmonary disease (COPD)	4 litres per minute	28% Venturi mask or patient's own mask
Exacerbation of cystic fibrosis	4 litres per minute	**NB** If respiratory rate is >30 breaths/min using Venturi mask set flow rate to 50% above the minimum specified for the mask.
Chronic neuromuscular disorders Chest wall disorders Morbid obesity (body mass index >40 kg/m²)	4 litres per minute	28% Venturi mask or patient's own mask
	5–10 litres per minute	Simple face mask

NB If the oxygen saturation remains below 88% change to simple face mask.

Oxygen

OXG

Controlled or low-dose supplemental oxygen for adults with COPD and other conditions requiring controlled or low-dose oxygen therapy

Target saturation **88–92%**	Administer the initial oxygen dose until a reliable SpO$_2$ measurement is available, then adjust oxygen flow to aim for target saturation within the range of **88–92%** or **pre-specified range** detailed on the patient's alert card, as per the table below.
NB Critical illness **AND** COPD/or other risk factors for hypercapnia.	If a patient with COPD or other risk factors for hypercapnia sustains or develops critical illness/injury then a target saturation level of 94-98% should be aimed for, but if this results in decreased conscious level or decreased respiratory rate decrease the oxygen flow and aim for 88-92%

NB BTS guidance states that patients with COPD and other risk factors for hypercapnia should have the same initial target saturations as other critically ill patients pending the results of blood gas results after which these patients may need controlled oxygen therapy with target range 88–92 or supported ventilation and/or hypercapnia with respiratory acidosis

Patients over 50 years of age who are long-term smokers with a history of exertional breathlessness and no other known cause of breathlessness should be treated as if having COPD.

*see Medicines: Best Practice checklist

MEDS

Oxygen

OXG

To supplemental oxygen required for adults with these conditions unless the patient is hypoxaemic but patients should be monitored closely

Target saturation 94–98%

If hypoxaemic (SpO$_2$ <94%) administer the initial oxygen dose, then adjust oxygen flow to aim for target saturation within the range of 94–98%, as per table below.

Condition	Initial dose	Method of administration
Myocardial infarction and acute coronary syndromes Stroke Cardiac rhythm disturbance Non-traumatic chest pain/discomfort Implantable cardioverter defibrillator firing Pregnancy and obstetric emergencies: – birth imminent – haemorrhage during pregnancy – pregnancy-induced hypertension – vaginal bleeding Abdominal pain Headache Hyperventilation syndrome or dysfunctional breathing	**SpO$_2$ <85%** 10–15 litres per minute	High concentration oxygen mask
	SpO$_2$ ≥85–93% 2–6 litres per minute	Nasal cannulae
	SpO$_2$ ≥94% 5–10 litres per minute	Simple face mask

185

Oxygen OXG

No supplemental oxygen required for adults with these conditions unless the patient is hypoxaemic but patients should be monitored closely

Target saturation 94–98%	If hypoxaemic (SpO$_2$ <94%) administer the initial oxygen dose, then adjust oxygen flow to aim for target saturation within the range of 94–98%, as per table below.		
Condition		**Initial dose**	**Method of administration**
• Most poisonings and drug overdoses (refer to Controlled or low-dose supplemental oxygen for adults with COPD and other conditions requiring controlled or low-dose oxygen therapy for **carbon monoxide poisoning** and special cases below for **paraquat or bleomycin poisoning**)		**SpO$_2$ <85%** 10–15 litres per minute	High concentration oxygen mask
• Metabolic and renal disorders • Acute and sub-acute neurological and muscular conditions producing muscle weakness (assess the need for assisted ventilation if **SpO$_2$ <94%**)		**SpO$_2$ ≥85–93%** 2–6 litres per minute	Nasal cannulae
• Post convulsion • Gastrointestinal bleeds • Glycaemic emergencies • Heat exhaustion/heat stroke		**SpO$_2$ ≥85–93%** 5–10 litres per minute	Simple face mask

*see Medicines: Best Practice checklist

MEDS

Oxygen

OXG

No supplemental oxygen required for adults with these conditions unless the patient is hypoxaemic but patients should be monitored closely

Target saturation	
94–98%	If hypoxaemic (SpO$_2$ <94%) administer the initial oxygen dose, then adjust oxygen flow to aim for target saturation within the range of 94–98%, as per table below.

Condition
SPECIAL CASES
• Poisoning with paraquat
• Poisoning with bleomycin

Initial dose	Method of administration
SpO$_2$ <85% 10-15 litres per minute	High concentration oxygen mask
SpO$_2$ ≥85–93% 2–6 litres per minute	Nasal cannulae
SpO$_2$ ≥85–93% 5–10 litres per minute	Simple face mask

NOTE – patients with **paraquat or bleomycin** poisoning may be harmed by supplemental oxygen so avoid oxygen unless the patient is hypoxaemic. Target saturation 85–88%.

*see Medicines: Best Practice checklist **MEDS**

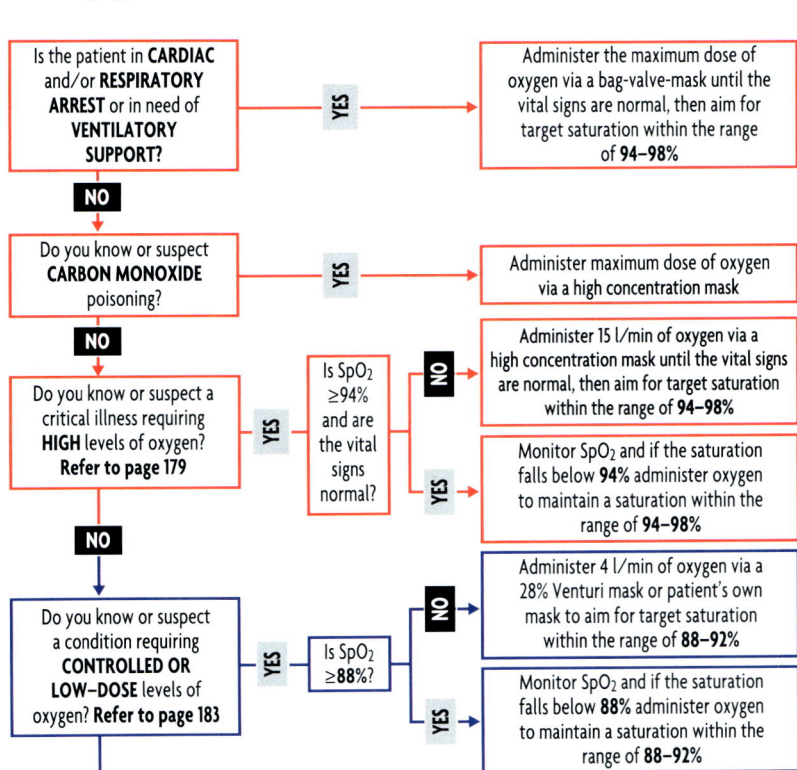

Oxygen   # OXG

Is the patient in **CARDIAC** and/or **RESPIRATORY ARREST** or in need of **VENTILATORY SUPPORT?**

YES → Administer the maximum dose of oxygen via a bag-valve-mask until the vital signs are normal, then aim for target saturation within the range of **94–98%**

NO

Do you know or suspect **CARBON MONOXIDE** poisoning?

YES → Administer maximum dose of oxygen via a high concentration mask

NO

Do you know or suspect a critical illness requiring **HIGH** levels of oxygen? **Refer to page 179**

YES → Is SpO_2 ≥94% and are the vital signs normal?

NO → Administer 15 l/min of oxygen via a high concentration mask until the vital signs are normal, then aim for target saturation within the range of **94–98%**

YES → Monitor SpO_2 and if the saturation falls below **94%** administer oxygen to maintain a saturation within the range of **94–98%**

NO

Do you know or suspect a condition requiring **CONTROLLED OR LOW-DOSE** levels of oxygen? **Refer to page 183**

YES → Is SpO_2 ≥**88%**?

NO → Administer 4 l/min of oxygen via a 28% Venturi mask or patient's own mask to aim for target saturation within the range of **88–92%**

YES → Monitor SpO_2 and if the saturation falls below **88%** administer oxygen to maintain a saturation within the range of **88–92%**

Oxygen OXG

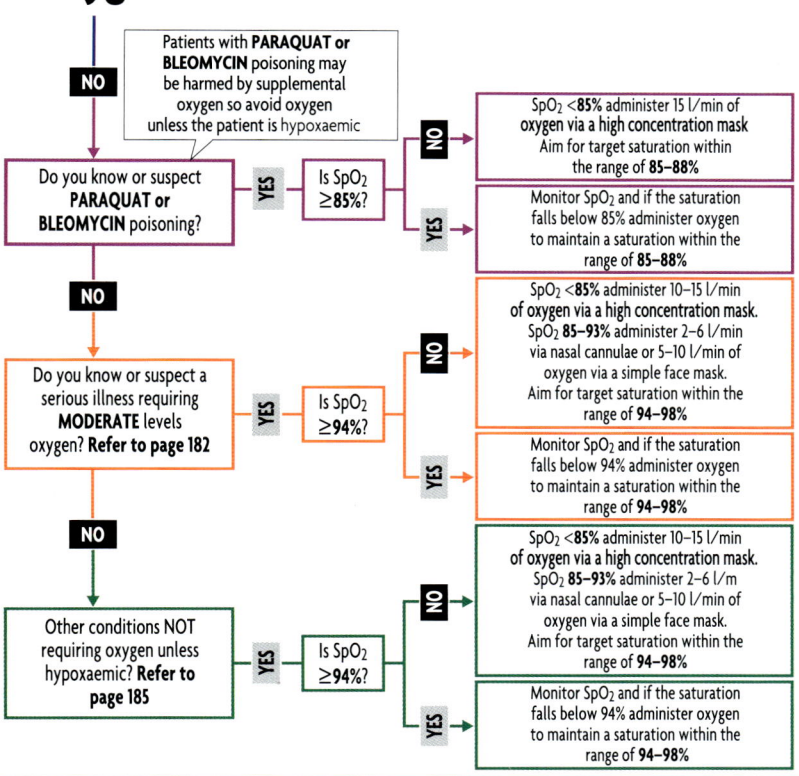

NO → Patients with **PARAQUAT or BLEOMYCIN** poisoning may be harmed by supplemental oxygen so avoid oxygen unless the patient is hypoxaemic

Do you know or suspect PARAQUAT or BLEOMYCIN poisoning?
- **YES** → Is SpO₂ ≥85%?
  - **NO** → SpO₂ <85% administer 15 l/min of **oxygen via a high concentration mask** Aim for target saturation within the range of **85–88%**
  - **YES** → Monitor SpO₂ and if the saturation falls below 85% administer oxygen to maintain a saturation within the range of **85–88%**
- **NO** ↓

Do you know or suspect a serious illness requiring MODERATE levels oxygen? Refer to page 182
- **YES** → Is SpO₂ ≥94%?
  - **NO** → SpO₂ <**85%** administer 10–15 l/min **of oxygen via a high concentration mask**. SpO₂ **85–93%** administer 2–6 l/min via nasal cannulae or 5–10 l/min of oxygen via a simple face mask. Aim for target saturation within the range of **94–98%**
  - **YES** → Monitor SpO₂ and if the saturation falls below 94% administer oxygen to maintain a saturation within the range of **94–98%**
- **NO** ↓

Other conditions NOT requiring oxygen unless hypoxaemic? Refer to page 185
- **YES** → Is SpO₂ ≥94%?
  - **NO** → SpO₂ <**85%** administer 10–15 l/min **of oxygen via a high concentration mask**. SpO₂ **85–93%** administer 2–6 l/m via nasal cannulae or 5–10 l/min of oxygen via a simple face mask. Aim for target saturation within the range of **94–98%**
  - **YES** → Monitor SpO₂ and if the saturation falls below 94% administer oxygen to maintain a saturation within the range of **94–98%**

see Medicines: Best Practice checklist **MEDS**

Paracetamol   PAR

Presentation

Both oral and intravenous preparations are available.

Oral

Paracetamol solutions/suspensions:

- **Infant paracetamol suspension** (120 milligrams in 5 ml), used from 3 months to 5 years.
- **Paracetamol 6 plus suspension** (250 milligrams in 5 ml), used from 6 years of age upwards.

Paracetamol tablets

- 500 milligram tablets (tablets may be broken in half).

Intravenous

- Bottle containing paracetamol 1 gram in 100 ml (10 mg/ml) for intravenous infusion for adults, adolescents and children weighing more than 33kg.
- Bottle containing paracetamol 500 milligrams in 50ml (10mg/ml) for intravenous infusion for term newborn, infants, toddlers and children weighing less than 33kg.

Indications

Oral

Relief of mild to moderate pain or high temperature with discomfort (not for high temperature alone).

Intravenous

As part of a balanced analgesic regimen for severe pain paracetamol is effective in reducing opioid requirements while improving analgesic efficacy and is an alternative analgesic when morphine is contraindicated.

Paracetamol   PAR

Actions
Analgesic (pain relieving) and antipyretic (temperature reducing) drug.

Contra-indications
Known paracetamol allergy.

Do **NOT** give further paracetamol if a paracetamol-containing product (e.g. Calpol, co-codamol) has already been given within the last 4 hours (6 hours in patients with renal impairment) or if the maximum cumulative daily dose has already been given.

Cautions
Take care when administering paracetamol injection to avoid dosing errors due to confusion between milligram (mg) and millilitre (mL), which could result in accidental overdose and death. Before administering, check when paracetamol was last administered and the cumulative paracetamol dose over the previous 24 hours.

The intravenous preparations come in different sizes, and due to the small amounts that are recommended for children from birth upwards, and for patients that weigh less than 50kg, extreme vigilance is needed. Refer to local procedure and guidance on how to administer dependant on what preparations are available to you.

Side Effects
Side effects are extremely rare; occasionally intravenous paracetamol may cause hypotension if administered too rapidly.

*see Medicines: Best Practice checklist   **MEDS**

Paracetamol   **PAR**

Additional Information

A febrile child should always be conveyed to hospital except where:

- a full assessment has been carried out,

and

- the child has no apparent serious underlying illness,

and

- the child has a defined clinical pathway for reassessment and follow up, with the full consent of the parent (or carer).

Paracetamol injection is supplied in plastic and glass containers. If a glass container is used it should be remembered that close monitoring is needed at the end of the infusion to avoid air embolism.

Paracetamol is not recommended for patients with cardiac chest pain.

Paracetamol PAR
Dosage and Administration

Ensure that:

1. Paracetamol (or an alternative paracetamol-containing product) has not been taken within the previous 4 hours (6 hours in renal impairment).
2. The maximum cumulative daily dose has not already been taken.
3. When administering to children, the correct paracetamol-containing solution/suspension for that patient's age is being used, i.e. 'infant paracetamol suspension' for those aged 0–5 years and 'paracetamol 6 plus suspension' for ages 6 years and over.

Route: Oral — infant paracetamol suspension (i.e. ages 3 months – 5 years).

AGE	INITIAL DOSE	REPEAT DOSE	DOSE INTERVAL	VOLUME	MAXIMUM DOSE
Adult	N/A	N/A	N/A	N/A	N/A
11 years	N/A	N/A	N/A	N/A	N/A
10 years	N/A	N/A	N/A	N/A	N/A
9 years	N/A	N/A	N/A	N/A	N/A
8 years	N/A	N/A	N/A	N/A	N/A
7 years	N/A	N/A	N/A	N/A	N/A
6 years	N/A	N/A	N/A	N/A	N/A
5 years 120 milligrams in 5 ml	240 milligrams	240 milligrams	4–6 hours	10 ml	960 milligrams in 24 hours

*see Medicines: Best Practice checklist **MEDS**

Paracetamol   **PAR**

Route: Oral – infant paracetamol suspension – *continued.*

AGE	INITIAL DOSE	REPEAT DOSE	DOSE INTERVAL	VOLUME	MAXIMUM DOSE
4 years 120 milligrams in 5 ml	240 milligrams	240 milligrams	4–6 hours	10 ml	960 milligrams in 24 hours
3 years 120 milligrams in 5 ml	180 milligrams	180 milligrams	4–6 hours	7.5 ml	720 milligrams in 24 hours
2 years 120 milligrams in 5 ml	180 milligrams	180 milligrams	4–6 hours	7.5 ml	720 milligrams in 24 hours
18 months 120 milligrams in 5 ml	120 milligrams	120 milligrams	4–6 hours	5 ml	480 milligrams in 24 hours
12 months 120 milligrams in 5 ml	120 milligrams	120 milligrams	4–6 hours	5 ml	480 milligrams in 24 hours
9 months 120 milligrams in 5 ml	120 milligrams	120 milligrams	4–6 hours	5 ml	480 milligrams in 24 hours
6 months 120 milligrams in 5 ml	120 milligrams	120 milligrams	4–6 hours	5 ml	480 milligrams in 24 hours
3 months 120 milligrams in 5 ml	60 milligrams	60 milligrams	4–6 hours	2.5 ml	240 milligrams in 24 hours
1 month	N/A	N/A	N/A	N/A	N/A
Birth	N/A	N/A	N/A	N/A	N/A

Paracetamol — PAR

Ensure that:
1. Paracetamol (or an alternative paracetamol-containing product) has not been taken within the previous 4 hours (6 hours in renal impairment).
2. The maximum cumulative daily dose has not already been taken.
3. When administering to children, the correct paracetamol-containing solution/suspension for that patient's age is being used, i.e. 'infant paracetamol suspension' for those aged 0–5 years and 'paracetamol 6 plus suspension' for ages 6 years and over.

Route: Oral — paracetamol 6 plus suspension (i.e. ages 6 years and over).

AGE	INITIAL DOSE	REPEAT DOSE	DOSE INTERVAL	VOLUME	MAXIMUM DOSE
16 years – Adult AND **over** 50 kg 250 milligrams in 5ml	500 milligrams – 1 gram	500 milligrams – 1 gram	4–6 hours	10–20 ml	2–4 grams in 24 hours
12–15 years OR 50 kg and **under** 250 milligrams in 5ml	500–750 milligrams	500–750 milligrams	4–6 hours	10–15 ml	2–3 grams in 24 hours

*see Medicines: Best Practice checklist **MEDS**

Paracetamol   **PAR**

Route: Oral – paracetamol 6 plus suspension – *continued*.

AGE	INITIAL DOSE	REPEAT DOSE	DOSE INTERVAL	VOLUME	MAXIMUM DOSE
11 years 250 milligrams in 5 ml	500 milligrams	500 milligrams	4–6 hours	10 ml	2 grams in 24 hours
10 years 250 milligrams in 5 ml	500 milligrams	500 milligrams	4–6 hours	10 ml	2 grams in 24 hours
9 years 250 milligrams in 5 ml	375 milligrams	375 milligrams	4–6 hours	7.5 ml	1.5 grams in 24 hours
8 years 250 milligrams in 5 ml	375 milligrams	375 milligrams	4–6 hours	7.5 ml	1.5 grams in 24 hours
7 years 250 milligrams in 5 ml	250 milligrams	250 milligrams	4–6 hours	5 ml	1 gram in 24 hours
6 years 250 milligrams in 5 ml	250 milligrams	250 milligrams	4–6 hours	5 ml	1 gram in 24 hours
5 years	N/A	N/A	N/A	N/A	N/A
4 years	N/A	N/A	N/A	N/A	N/A
3 years	N/A	N/A	N/A	N/A	N/A
2 years	N/A	N/A	N/A	N/A	N/A
18 months	N/A	N/A	N/A	N/A	N/A
12 months	N/A	N/A	N/A	N/A	N/A
9 months	N/A	N/A	N/A	N/A	N/A

Paracetamol   PAR

AGE	INITIAL DOSE	REPEAT DOSE	DOSE INTERVAL	VOLUME	MAXIMUM DOSE
6 months	N/A	N/A	N/A	N/A	N/A
3 months	N/A	N/A	N/A	N/A	N/A
1 month	N/A	N/A	N/A	N/A	N/A
Birth	N/A	N/A	N/A	N/A	N/A

Ensure that:

1. Paracetamol (or an alternative paracetamol-containing product) has not been taken within the previous 4 hours (6 hours in renal impairment).
2. The maximum cumulative daily dose has not already been taken.

Route: Oral – tablet.

AGE	INITIAL DOSE	REPEAT DOSE	DOSE INTERVAL	VOLUME	MAXIMUM DOSE
16 years – Adult AND **over** 50 kg 500 milligrams per tablet	500 milligrams – 1 gram	500 milligrams – 1 gram	4–6 hours	1–2 tablets	2–4 grams in 24 hours
12 years – 15 years OR 50 kg and **under** 500 milligrams per tablet	500–750 milligrams	500–750 milligrams	4–6 hours	1–1.5 tablets	2–3 grams in 24 hours

*see Medicines: Best Practice checklist **MEDS**

Paracetamol   PAR

Ensure that:
1. Paracetamol (or an alternative paracetamol-containing product) has not been taken within the previous 4 hours (6 hours in renal impairment).
2. The maximum cumulative daily dose has not already been taken.
3. IV paracetamol is only used when managing **severe pain** (use an oral preparation when managing fever with discomfort).

Route: Intravenous infusion; given over 15 minutes.

AGE	INITIAL DOSE	REPEAT DOSE	DOSE INTERVAL	VOLUME	MAXIMUM DOSE
12 years – Adult AND **over** 50 kg 10 milligrams in 1ml	1 gram	1 gram	4–6 hours	100 ml	4 grams in 24 hours
12 years – Adult AND **under** 50 kg 10 milligrams in 1ml	750 milligrams	750 milligrams	4–6 hours	75 ml	3 grams in 24 hours
11 years 10 milligrams in 1 ml	500 milligrams	500 milligrams	4–6 hours	50 ml	2 grams in 24 hours

Paracetamol PAR

Route: Intravenous infusion; given over 15 minutes – *continued*.

AGE	INITIAL DOSE	REPEAT DOSE	DOSE INTERVAL	VOLUME	MAXIMUM DOSE
10 years 10 milligrams in 1 ml	500 milligrams	500 milligrams	4–6 hours	50 ml	2 grams in 24 hours
9 years 10 milligrams in 1 ml	450 milligrams	450 milligrams	4–6 hours	45 ml	1.8 grams in 24 hours
8 years 10 milligrams in 1 ml	400 milligrams	400 milligrams	4–6 hours	40 ml	1.6 grams in 24 hours
7 years 10 milligrams in 1 ml	350 milligrams	350 milligrams	4–6 hours	35 ml	1.4 grams in 24 hours
6 years 10 milligrams in 1 ml	300 milligrams	300 milligrams	4–6 hours	30 ml	1.2 grams in 24 hours
5 years 10 milligrams in 1 ml	300 milligrams	300 milligrams	4–6 hours	30 ml	1.2 gram in 24 hours
4 years 10 milligrams in 1 ml	250 milligrams	250 milligrams	4–6 hours	25 ml	1 gram in 24 hours
3 years 10 milligrams in 1 ml	200 milligrams	200 milligrams	4–6 hours	20 ml	800 milligrams in 24 hours

*see Medicines: Best Practice checklist **MEDS**

Paracetamol   **PAR**

Route: Intravenous infusion; given over 15 minutes − *continued*.

AGE	INITIAL DOSE	REPEAT DOSE	DOSE INTERVAL	VOLUME	MAXIMUM DOSE
2 years 10 milligrams in 1 ml	200 milligrams	200 milligrams	4−6 hours	20 ml	800 milligrams in 24 hours
18 months 10 milligrams in 1 ml	150 milligrams	150 milligrams	4−6 hours	15 ml	600 milligrams in 24 hours
12 months 10 milligrams in 1 ml	150 milligrams	150 milligrams	4−6 hours	15 ml	600 milligrams in 24 hours
9 months 10 milligrams in 1 ml	90 milligrams	90 milligrams	4−6 hours	9 ml	270 milligrams in 24 hours
6 months 10 milligrams in 1 ml	80 milligrams	80 milligrams	4−6 hours	8 ml	240 milligrams in 24 hours
3 months 10 milligrams in 1 ml	60 milligrams	60 milligrams	4−6 hours	6 ml	180 milligrams in 24 hours
1 month 10 milligrams in 1 ml	45 milligrams	45 milligrams	4−6 hours	4.5 ml	135 milligrams in 24 hours
Birth 10 milligrams in 1 ml	35 milligrams	35 milligrams	4−6 hours	3.5 ml	105 milligrams in 24 hours

Salbutamol SLB

Presentation
Nebules containing salbutamol 2.5 milligrams/ 2.5 ml or 5 milligrams/2.5 ml.

Indications
Acute asthma attack where normal inhaler therapy has failed to relieve symptoms.

Expiratory wheezing associated with allergy, anaphylaxis, beta-blocker overdose, smoke inhalation or other lower airway cause.

Exacerbation of chronic obstructive pulmonary disease (COPD).

Actions
Salbutamol is a selective $beta_2$ adrenoreceptor stimulant drug. This has a relaxant effect on the smooth muscle in the medium and smaller airways, which are in spasm in acute asthma attacks. If given by nebuliser, especially if oxygen powered, its smooth-muscle relaxing action, combined with the airway moistening effect of nebulisation, can relieve the attack rapidly.

Contra-indications
None in the emergency situation.

*see Medicines: Best Practice checklist **MEDS**

Salbutamol   SLB

Cautions

Salbutamol should be used with care in patients with:

- Hypertension
- Angina
- Overactive thyroid
- Late pregnancy (can relax uterus)
- Bronchomalacia / laryngomalacia / tracheomalacia (abnormal softening of the bronchial tubes, larynx and trachea)
- Severe hypertension may occur in patients on beta-blockers and half doses should be used unless there is profound hypotension

If COPD is a possibility limit nebulisation with oxygen to 6 minutes.

Side Effects

Tremor (shaking).

Tachycardia.

Palpitations.

Headache.

Feeling of tension.

Peripheral vasodilatation.

Muscle cramps.

Rash.

Salbutamol SLB

Additional Information

In acute severe or life-threatening asthma ipratropium should be given after the first dose of salbutamol. In acute asthma or COPD unresponsive to salbutamol alone, a single dose of ipratropium may be given after salbutamol.

Salbutamol often provides initial relief. In more severe attacks, however, the use of steroids by injection or orally and further nebuliser therapy will be required. Do not be lulled into a false sense of security by an initial improvement after salbutamol nebulisation.

Nebules should be protected from light after removal from the foil overwrap pouch. They should be disposed of after a reduced period of expiry, indicated on the pouch.

Salbutamol is not indicated in bronchiolitis. It will not benefit the condition and the resultant tachycardia may confuse subsequent clinical assessment in hospital.

Dosage and Administration

- **In life-threatening or acute severe asthma:** undertake a **TIME CRITICAL** transfer to the **NEAREST SUITABLE RECEIVING HOSPITAL** and provide nebulisation en-route.
- If COPD is a possibility limit nebulisation with oxygen to 6 minutes.
- The pulse rate in children may exceed 140 after significant doses of salbutamol; this is not usually of any clinical significance and should not usually preclude further use of the drug.

*see Medicines: Best Practice checklist   **MEDS**

Salbutamol   **SLB**

● Repeat doses should be discontinued if the side effects are becoming significant (e.g. tremors, tachycardia >140 beats per minute in adults) – this is a clinical decision by the ambulance clinician.

Route: Nebulised with 6–8 litres per minute of oxygen.

AGE	INITIAL DOSE	REPEAT DOSE	DOSE INTERVAL	VOLUME	MAX DOSE
Adult 2.5 milligrams in 2.5 ml	5 milligrams	5 milligrams	5 minutes	5 ml	No limit

Route: Nebulised with 6–8 litres per minute of oxygen.

AGE	INITIAL DOSE	REPEAT DOSE	DOSE INTERVAL	VOLUME	MAX DOSE
Adult 5 milligrams in 2.5 ml	5 milligrams	5 milligrams	5 minutes	2.5 ml	No limit

Sodium Chloride 0.9% SCP

Presentation
100 ml, 250 ml, 500 ml and 1,000 ml packs of sodium chloride intravenous infusion 0.9%.

5 ml and 10 ml ampoules for use as flushes.

5 ml and 10 ml pre-loaded syringes for use as flushes.

Indications

Adult fluid therapy
- Medical conditions without haemorrhage.
- Medical conditions with haemorrhage.
- Trauma related haemorrhage.
- Burns.
- Limb crush injury.

Child fluid therapy
- Medical conditions.
- Trauma related haemorrhage.
- Burns.

Flush
- As a flush to confirm patency of an intravenous or intraosseous cannula.
- As a flush following drug administration.

*see Medicines: Best Practice checklist   **MEDS**

Sodium Chloride 0.9%   **SCP**

Actions

Increases vascular fluid volume which consequently raises cardiac output and improves perfusion.

Contra-Indications

Soduim Chloride should **NOT** be administered solely for the purposes of keeping a vein open (TKO/TKVO) as this may lead to inadvertent excess fluid administration.

Side Effects

Over-infusion may precipitate pulmonary oedema and cause breathlessness.

Additional Information

Fluid replacement in cases of dehydration should occur over hours; rapid fluid replacement is seldom indicated; **refer to Intravascular Fluid Therapy**.

Dosage and Administration

Route: Intravenous or intraosseous for **ALL** conditions.

FLUSH

AGE	INITIAL DOSE	REPEAT DOSE	DOSE INTERVAL	VOLUME	MAXIMUM DOSE
Adult 0.9%	2 ml – 5 ml	2 ml – 5 ml	PRN	2 – 5 ml	N/A
Adult 0.9%	10 ml – 20 ml (if infusing glucose)	10 ml – 20 ml (if infusing glucose)	PRN	10 – 20 ml	N/A

Sodium Chloride 0.9% — SCP

ADULT MEDICAL EMERGENCIES

General medical conditions without haemorrhage: Anaphylaxis, hyperglycaemic ketoacidosis

AGE	INITIAL DOSE	REPEAT DOSE	DOSE INTERVAL	VOLUME	MAXIMUM DOSE
Adult 0.9%	250 ml	250 ml	PRN	**250 ml**	2 litres

Sepsis: Clinical signs of infection **AND** systolic BP<90 mmHg

AGE	INITIAL DOSE	REPEAT DOSE	DOSE INTERVAL	VOLUME	MAXIMUM DOSE
Adult 0.9%	500 ml	Repeat ONCE if hypotensive	15 minutes	**500 ml**	2 litres

Diabetic Ketoacidosis (DKA)

AGE	INITIAL DOSE	REPEAT DOSE	DOSE INTERVAL	VOLUME	MAXIMUM DOSE
Adult 18 years and over 0.9%	500 ml	500 ml	PRN	**500 ml**	1 litre

*see Medicines: Best Practice checklist **MEDS**

Sodium Chloride 0.9%   **SCP**

Medical conditions with haemorrhage: Systolic BP<90 mmHg and signs of poor perfusion

AGE	INITIAL DOSE	REPEAT DOSE	DOSE INTERVAL	VOLUME	MAXIMUM DOSE
Adult 0.9%	250 ml	250 ml	PRN	250 ml	2 litres

ADULT TRAUMA EMERGENCIES

Blunt trauma, head trauma or penetrating limb trauma: The general aim of fluid therapy is to maintain a palpable peripheral pulse (radial) OR systolic BP of 90mmHg.

AGE	INITIAL DOSE	REPEAT DOSE	DOSE INTERVAL	VOLUME	MAXIMUM DOSE
Adult 0.9%	250 ml	250 ml	PRN	250 ml	2 litres

Penetrating torso trauma: The general aim of fluid therapy is to maintain a palpable peripheral pulse (radial) OR systolic BP of 90mmHg.

AGE	INITIAL DOSE	REPEAT DOSE	DOSE INTERVAL	VOLUME	MAXIMUM DOSE
Adult 0.9%	250 ml	250 ml	PRN	250 ml	2 litres

Sodium Chloride 0.9% SCP

Burns:

- Total body surface area (TBSA): between 15% and 25% and time to hospital is greater than 30 minutes
- TBSA: more than 25%

AGE	INITIAL DOSE	REPEAT DOSE	DOSE INTERVAL	VOLUME	MAXIMUM DOSE
Adult 0.9%	1 litre	NONE	N/A	1 litre	1 litre

Crush syndrome

AGE	INITIAL DOSE	REPEAT DOSE	DOSE INTERVAL	VOLUME	MAXIMUM DOSE
Adult 0.9%	2 litres	NONE	N/A	2 litres	2 litres

NB Manage crush injury of the torso as per blunt trauma.

*see Medicines: Best Practice checklist **MEDS**

Sodium Chloride 0.9%   **SCP**

MEDICAL EMERGENCIES IN CHILDREN (20 ml/kg)
NB Exceptions: cardiac failure, renal failure, diabetic ketoacidosis
(see following).

AGE	INITIAL DOSE	REPEAT DOSE	DOSE INTERVAL	VOLUME	MAXIMUM DOSE
11 years 0.9%	500 ml	500 ml	PRN	500 ml	1,000 ml
10 years 0.9%	500 ml	500 ml	PRN	500 ml	1,000 ml
9 years 0.9%	500 ml	500 ml	PRN	500 ml	1,000 ml
8 years 0.9%	500 ml	500 ml	PRN	500 ml	1,000 ml
7 years 0.9%	460 ml	460 ml	PRN	460 ml	920 ml
6 years 0.9%	420 ml	420 ml	PRN	420 ml	840 ml
5 years 0.9%	380 ml	380 ml	PRN	380 ml	760 ml
4 years 0.9%	320 ml	320 ml	PRN	320 ml	640 ml
3 years 0.9%	280 ml	280 ml	PRN	280 ml	560 ml
2 years 0.9%	240 ml	240 ml	PRN	240 ml	480 ml
18 months 0.9%	220 ml	220 ml	PRN	220 ml	440 ml

Sodium Chloride 0.9% SCP

MEDICAL EMERGENCIES IN CHILDREN (20 ml/kg) – *continued*.
NB Exceptions: cardiac failure, renal failure, diabetic ketoacidosis (see following).

AGE	INITIAL DOSE	REPEAT DOSE	DOSE INTERVAL	VOLUME	MAXIMUM DOSE
12 months 0.9%	200 ml	200 ml	PRN	200 ml	400 ml
9 months 0.9%	180 ml	180 ml	PRN	180 ml	360 ml
6 months 0.9%	160 ml	160 ml	PRN	160 ml	320 ml
3 months 0.9%	120 ml	120 ml	PRN	120 ml	240 ml
1 month 0.9%	90 ml	90 ml	PRN	90 ml	180 ml
Birth 0.9%	70 ml	70 ml	PRN	70 ml	140 ml

*see Medicines: Best Practice checklist **MEDS**

Sodium Chloride 0.9%

SCP

MEDICAL EMERGENCIES IN CHILDREN
Heart failure or renal failure (10 ml/kg)

AGE	INITIAL DOSE	REPEAT DOSE	DOSE INTERVAL	VOLUME	MAXIMUM DOSE
11 years 0.9%	350 ml	350 ml	PRN	350 ml	1,000 ml
10 years 0.9%	320 ml	320 ml	PRN	320 ml	1,000 ml
9 years 0.9%	290 ml	290 ml	PRN	290 ml	1,000 ml
8 years 0.9%	250 ml	250 ml	PRN	250 ml	1,000 ml
7 years 0.9%	230 ml	230 ml	PRN	230 ml	920 ml
6 years 0.9%	210 ml	210 ml	PRN	210 ml	840 ml
5 years 0.9%	190 ml	190 ml	PRN	190 ml	760 ml
4 years 0.9%	160 ml	160 ml	PRN	160 ml	640 ml
3 years 0.9%	140 ml	140 ml	PRN	140 ml	560 ml
2 years 0.9%	120 ml	120 ml	PRN	120 ml	480 ml
18 months 0.9%	110 ml	110 ml	PRN	110 ml	440 ml

Sodium Chloride 0.9% — SCP

MEDICAL EMERGENCIES IN CHILDREN.
Heart failure or renal failure (10 ml/kg) – *continued.*

AGE	INITIAL DOSE	REPEAT DOSE	DOSE INTERVAL	VOLUME	MAXIMUM DOSE
12 months 0.9%	100 ml	100 ml	PRN	100 ml	400 ml
9 months 0.9%	90 ml	90 ml	PRN	90 ml	360 ml
6 months 0.9%	80 ml	80 ml	PRN	80 ml	320 ml
3 months 0.9%	60 ml	60 ml	PRN	60 ml	240 ml
1 month 0.9%	45 ml	45 ml	PRN	45 ml	180 ml
Birth 0.9%	35 ml	35 ml	PRN	35 ml	140 ml

*see Medicines: Best Practice checklist · **MEDS**

Sodium Chloride 0.9%   **SCP**

MEDICAL EMERGENCIES IN CHILDREN
Diabetic ketoacidosis (10 ml/kg) administer **ONCE** only over 15 minutes.

AGE	INITIAL DOSE	REPEAT DOSE	DOSE INTERVAL	VOLUME	MAXIMUM DOSE
11 years 0.9%	350 ml	NONE	NA	350 ml	350 ml
10 years 0.9%	320 ml	NONE	NA	320 ml	320 ml
9 years 0.9%	290 ml	NONE	NA	290 ml	290 ml
8 years 0.9%	250 ml	NONE	NA	250 ml	250 ml
7 years 0.9%	230 ml	NONE	NA	230 ml	230 ml
6 years 0.9%	210 ml	NONE	NA	210 ml	210 ml
5 years 0.9%	190 ml	NONE	NA	190 ml	190 ml
4 years 0.9%	160 ml	NONE	NA	160 ml	160 ml
3 years 0.9%	140 ml	NONE	NA	140 ml	140 ml
2 years 0.9%	120 ml	NONE	NA	120 ml	120 ml
18 months 0.9%	110 ml	NONE	NA	110 ml	110 ml

Sodium Chloride 0.9% SCP

MEDICAL EMERGENCIES IN CHILDREN.
Diabetic ketoacidosis (10 ml/kg) administer **ONCE** only over 15 minutes – *continued.*

AGE	INITIAL DOSE	REPEAT DOSE	DOSE INTERVAL	VOLUME	MAXIMUM DOSE
12 months 0.9%	100 ml	NONE	NA	100 ml	100 ml
9 months 0.9%	90 ml	NONE	NA	90 ml	90 ml
6 months 0.9%	80 ml	NONE	NA	80 ml	80 ml
3 months 0.9%	60 ml	NONE	NA	60 ml	60 ml
1 month 0.9%	45 ml	NONE	NA	45 ml	45 ml
Birth 0.9%	35 ml	NONE	NA	35 ml	35 ml

*see Medicines: Best Practice checklist **MEDS**

Sodium Chloride 0.9% **SCP**

TRAUMA EMERGENCIES IN CHILDREN (5 ml/kg)[a]

NB Exceptions: burns.

AGE	INITIAL DOSE	REPEAT DOSE	DOSE INTERVAL	VOLUME	MAXIMUM DOSE
11 years 0.9%	175 ml	175 ml	PRN	175 ml	1,000 ml
10 years 0.9%	160 ml	160 ml	PRN	160 ml	1,000 ml
9 years 0.9%	145 ml	145 ml	PRN	145 ml	1,000 ml
8 years 0.9%	130 ml	130 ml	PRN	130 ml	1,000 ml
7 years 0.9%	115 ml	115 ml	PRN	115 ml	920 ml
6 years 0.9%	105 ml	105 ml	PRN	105 ml	840 ml
5 years 0.9%	95 ml	95 ml	PRN	95 ml	760 ml
4 years 0.9%	80 ml	80 ml	PRN	80 ml	640 ml
3 years 0.9%	70 ml	70 ml	PRN	70 ml	560 ml
2 years 0.9%	60 ml	60 ml	PRN	60 ml	480 ml
18 months 0.9%	55 ml	55 ml	PRN	55 ml	440 ml

Sodium Chloride 0.9% SCP

TRAUMA EMERGENCIES IN CHILDREN (5 ml/kg) *continued.*

NB Exceptions: burns.

AGE	INITIAL DOSE	REPEAT DOSE	DOSE INTERVAL	VOLUME	MAXIMUM DOSE
12 months 0.9%	50 ml	50 ml	PRN	50 ml	400 ml
9 months 0.9%	45 ml	45 ml	PRN	45 ml	360 ml
6 months 0.9%	40 ml	40 ml	PRN	40 ml	320 ml
3 months 0.9%	30 ml	30 ml	PRN	30 ml	240 ml
1 month 0.9%	20 ml	20 ml	PRN	20 ml	180 ml
Birth 0.9%	20 ml	20 ml	PRN	20 ml	140 ml

[a]Seek advice to exceed maximum dose in trauma.

*see Medicines: Best Practice checklist **MEDS**

Sodium Chloride 0.9%   **SCP**

Burns (10 ml/kg, given over 1 hour):
- TBSA: between 10% and 20% and time to hospital is greater than 30 minutes
- TBSA: more than 20%

AGE	INITIAL DOSE	REPEAT DOSE	DOSE INTERVAL	VOLUME	MAXIMUM DOSE
11 years 0.9%	350 ml	NONE	N/A	350 ml	350 ml
10 years 0.9%	320 ml	NONE	N/A	320 ml	320 ml
9 years 0.9%	290 ml	NONE	N/A	290 ml	290 ml
8 years 0.9%	250 ml	NONE	N/A	250 ml	250 ml
7 years 0.9%	230 ml	NONE	N/A	230 ml	230 ml
6 years 0.9%	210 ml	NONE	N/A	210 ml	210 ml
5 years 0.9%	190 ml	NONE	N/A	190 ml	190 ml
4 years 0.9%	160 ml	NONE	N/A	160 ml	160 ml
3 years 0.9%	140 ml	NONE	N/A	140 ml	140 ml
2 years 0.9%	120 ml	NONE	N/A	120 ml	120 ml

Sodium Chloride 0.9%   SCP

Burns (10 ml/kg, given over 1 hour) *continued*.
- TBSA: between 10% and 20% and time to hospital is greater than 30 minutes
- TBSA: more than 20%.

AGE	INITIAL DOSE	REPEAT DOSE	DOSE INTERVAL	VOLUME	MAXIMUM DOSE
18 months 0.9%	110 ml	NONE	N/A	110 ml	110 ml
12 months 0.9%	100 ml	NONE	N/A	100 ml	100 ml
9 months 0.9%	90 ml	NONE	N/A	90 ml	90 ml
6 months 0.9%	80 ml	NONE	N/A	80 ml	80 ml
3 months 0.9%	60 ml	NONE	N/A	60 ml	60 ml
1 month 0.9%	45 ml	NONE	N/A	45 ml	45 ml
Birth 0.9%	35 ml	NONE	N/A	35 ml	35 ml

*see Medicines: Best Practice checklist

Sodium Lactate Compound · SLC

Presentation

250 ml, 500 ml and 1,000 ml packs of compound sodium lactate intravenous infusion (also called Hartmann's solution for injection or Ringer's lactate solution for injection).

Indications

Blood and fluid loss, to correct hypovolaemia and improve tissue perfusion if sodium chloride 0.9% is **NOT** available.

Dehydration.

Actions

Increases vascular fluid volume which consequently raises cardiac output and improves perfusion.

Contra-Indications

Diabetic hyperglycaemic ketoacidotic coma, and precoma.
NB Administer 0.9% sodium chloride intravenous infusion.

Neonates.

Cautions

Sodium lactate should not be used in limb crush injury when 0.9% sodium chloride is available.

Renal failure.

Liver failure.

Sodium Lactate Compound — SLC

Side Effects

Infusion of an excessive volume may overload the circulation and precipitate heart failure (increased breathlessness, wheezing and distended neck veins). Volume overload is unlikely if the patient is correctly assessed initially and it is very unlikely indeed if patient response is assessed after initial 250 ml infusion and then after each 250 ml of infusion. If there is evidence of this complication, the patient should be transported rapidly to nearest suitable receiving hospital whilst administering high-flow oxygen.

Do not administer further fluid.

Additional Information

Compound sodium lactate intravenous infusion contains mainly sodium, but also small amounts of potassium and lactate. It is useful for initial fluid replacement in cases of blood loss.

The volume of compound sodium lactate intravenous infusion needed is 3 times as great as the volume of blood loss. Sodium lactate has **NO** oxygen carrying capacity.

*see Medicines: Best Practice checklist **MEDS**

Sodium Lactate Compound   **SLC**

Dosage and Administration if sodium chloride 0.9% is NOT available.

Route: Intravenous or intraosseous for **ALL** conditions.

ADULT MEDICAL EMERGENCIES

General medical conditions without haemorrhage: anaphylaxis, dehydration*

NB Exception sodium lactate compound is contra-indicated in diabetic ketoacidosis – **refer to Sodium Chloride 0.9%**.

AGE	INITIAL DOSE	REPEAT DOSE	DOSE INTERVAL	VOLUME	MAXIMUM DOSE
Adult Compound	250 ml	250 ml	PRN	250 ml	1 litre

Sepsis: Clinical signs of infection **AND** systolic BP<90 mmHg **AND** tachypnoea

AGE	INITIAL DOSE	REPEAT DOSE	DOSE INTERVAL	VOLUME	MAXIMUM DOSE
Adult Compound	1 litre	1 litre	30 minutes	1 litre	2 litres

*In cases of dehydration fluid replacement should usually occur over hours.

Sodium Lactate Compound   SLC

ADULT TRAUMA EMERGENCIES

Medical conditions with haemorrhage: Systolic BP<90 mmHg and signs of poor perfusion

AGE	INITIAL DOSE	REPEAT DOSE	DOSE INTERVAL	VOLUME	MAXIMUM DOSE
Adult Compound	250 ml	250 ml	PRN	250 ml	2 litres

Blunt trauma, head trauma or penetrating limb trauma: Systolic BP<90 mmHg and signs of poor perfusion

AGE	INITIAL DOSE	REPEAT DOSE	DOSE INTERVAL	VOLUME	MAXIMUM DOSE
Adult Compound	250 ml	250 ml	PRN	250 ml	2 litres

Penetrating torso trauma: Systolic BP<60 mmHg and signs of poor perfusion

AGE	INITIAL DOSE	REPEAT DOSE	DOSE INTERVAL	VOLUME	MAXIMUM DOSE
Adult Compound	250 ml	250 ml	PRN	250 ml	2 litres

see Medicines: Best Practice checklist **MEDS**

Sodium Lactate Compound   **SLC**

Burns:
- TBSA: between 15% and 25% and time to hospital is greater than 30 minutes.
- TBSA: more than 25%.

AGE	INITIAL DOSE	REPEAT DOSE	DOSE INTERVAL	VOLUME	MAXIMUM DOSE
Adult Compound	1 litre	N/A	N/A	1 litre	1 litre

Limb crush injury

AGE	INITIAL DOSE	REPEAT DOSE	DOSE INTERVAL	VOLUME	MAXIMUM DOSE
Adult Compound	2 litres	N/A	N/A	2 litres	2 litres

NB Sodium chloride 0.9% is the fluid of choice in crush injury.
NB Manage crush injury of the torso as per blunt trauma.

Sodium Lactate Compound — SLC

MEDICAL EMERGENCIES IN CHILDREN (20 ml/kg)

NB Exceptions heart failure, renal failure, liver failure, diabetic ketoacidosis (sodium lactate compound is contra-indicated in diabetic ketoacidosis – **refer to Sodium Chloride 0.9%**).

AGE	INITIAL DOSE	REPEAT DOSE	DOSE INTERVAL	VOLUME	MAXIMUM DOSE
11 years Compound	500 ml	500 ml	PRN	500 ml	1 litre
10 years Compound	500 ml	500 ml	PRN	500 ml	1 litre
9 years Compound	500 ml	500 ml	PRN	500 ml	1 litre
8 years Compound	500 ml	500 ml	PRN	500 ml	1 litre
7 years Compound	460 ml	460 ml	PRN	460 ml	920 ml
6 years Compound	420 ml	420 ml	PRN	420 ml	840 ml
5 years Compound	380 ml	380 ml	PRN	380 ml	760 ml
4 years Compound	320 ml	320 ml	PRN	320 ml	640 ml
3 years Compound	280 ml	280 ml	PRN	280 ml	560 ml

*see Medicines: Best Practice checklist **MEDS**

Sodium Lactate Compound   **SLC**

MEDICAL EMERGENCIES IN CHILDREN (20 ml/kg) – *continued*.
NB Exceptions heart failure, renal failure, liver failure, diabetic
ketoacidosis (sodium lactate compound is contra-indicated in diabetic
ketoacidosis – **refer to Sodium Chloride 0.9%**).

AGE	INITIAL DOSE	REPEAT DOSE	DOSE INTERVAL	VOLUME	MAXIMUM DOSE
2 years Compound	240 ml	240 ml	PRN	240 ml	480 ml
18 months Compound	220 ml	220 ml	PRN	220 ml	440 ml
12 months Compound	200 ml	200 ml	PRN	200 ml	400 ml
9 months Compound	180 ml	180 ml	PRN	180 ml	360 ml
6 months Compound	160 ml	160 ml	PRN	160 ml	320 ml
3 months Compound	120 ml	120 ml	PRN	120 ml	240 ml
1 month Compound	90 ml	90 ml	PRN	90 ml	180 ml
Birth N/A	N/A	N/A	N/A	N/A	N/A

Sodium Lactate Compound — SLC

MEDICAL EMERGENCIES IN CHILDREN

Heart failure or renal failure (10 ml/kg)

AGE	INITIAL DOSE	REPEAT DOSE	DOSE INTERVAL	VOLUME	MAXIMUM DOSE
11 years Compound	350 ml	350 ml	PRN	350 ml	700 ml
10 years Compound	320 ml	320 ml	PRN	320 ml	640 ml
9 years Compound	290 ml	290 ml	PRN	290 ml	580 ml
8 years Compound	250 ml	250 ml	PRN	250 ml	500 ml
7 years Compound	230 ml	230 ml	PRN	230 ml	460 ml
6 years Compound	210 ml	210 ml	PRN	210 ml	420 ml
5 years Compound	190 ml	190 ml	PRN	190 ml	380 ml
4 years Compound	160 ml	160 ml	PRN	160 ml	320 ml
3 years Compound	140 ml	140 ml	PRN	140 ml	280 ml
2 years Compound	120 ml	120 ml	PRN	120 ml	240 ml

Sodium Lactate Compound

SLC

MEDICAL EMERGENCIES IN CHILDREN – continued.

Heart failure or renal failure (10 ml/kg).

AGE	INITIAL DOSE	REPEAT DOSE	DOSE INTERVAL	VOLUME	MAXIMUM DOSE
Birth	N/A	N/A	N/A	N/A	N/A
1 month Compound	45 ml	45 ml	PRN	45 ml	90 ml
3 months Compound	60 ml	60 ml	PRN	60 ml	120 ml
6 months Compound	80 ml	80 ml	PRN	80 ml	160 ml
9 months Compound	90 ml	90 ml	PRN	90 ml	180 ml
12 months Compound	100 ml	100 ml	PRN	100 ml	200 ml
18 months Compound	110 ml	110 ml	PRN	110 ml	220 ml

*see Medicines: Best Practice checklist

Sodium Lactate Compound   SLC

TRAUMA EMERGENCIES IN CHILDREN (5 ml/kg)

NB Exceptions: burns.

AGE	INITIAL DOSE	REPEAT DOSE	DOSE INTERVAL	VOLUME	MAXIMUM DOSE
11 years Compound	175 ml	175 ml	PRN	175 ml	1 litre
10 years Compound	160 ml	160 ml	PRN	160 ml	1 litre
9 years Compound	145 ml	145 ml	PRN	145 ml	1 litre
8 years Compound	130 ml	130 ml	PRN	130 ml	1 litre
7 years Compound	115 ml	115 ml	PRN	115 ml	920 ml
6 years Compound	105 ml	105 ml	PRN	105 ml	840 ml
5 years Compound	95 ml	95 ml	PRN	95 ml	760 ml
4 years Compound	80 ml	80 ml	PRN	80 ml	640 ml
3 years Compound	70 ml	70 ml	PRN	70 ml	560 ml
2 years Compound	60 ml	60 ml	PRN	60 ml	480 ml

Sodium Lactate Compound

SLC

TRAUMA EMERGENCIES IN CHILDREN (5 ml/kg) – *continued.*

NB Exceptions: burns.

AGE	INITIAL DOSE	REPEAT DOSE	DOSE INTERVAL	VOLUME	MAXIMUM DOSE
18 months Compound	55 ml	55 ml	PRN	55 ml	440 ml
12 months Compound	50 ml	50 ml	PRN	50 ml	400 ml
9 months Compound	45 ml	45 ml	PRN	45 ml	360 ml
6 months Compound	40 ml	40 ml	PRN	40 ml	320 ml
3 months Compound	30 ml	30 ml	PRN	30 ml	240 ml
1 month Compound	20 ml	20 ml	PRN	20 ml	180 ml
Birth	N/A	N/A	N/A	N/A	N/A

Sodium Lactate Compound — SLC

Burns (10 ml/kg, given over 1 hour):
- TBSA: between 10% and 20% and time to hospital is greater than 30 minutes.
- TBSA: more than 20%.

AGE	INITIAL DOSE	REPEAT DOSE	DOSE INTERVAL	VOLUME	MAXIMUM DOSE
11 years Compound	350 ml	NONE	N/A	350 ml	350 ml
10 years Compound	320 ml	NONE	N/A	320 ml	320 ml
9 years Compound	290 ml	NONE	N/A	290 ml	290 ml
8 years Compound	250 ml	NONE	N/A	250 ml	250 ml
7 years Compound	230 ml	NONE	N/A	230 ml	230 ml
6 years Compound	210 ml	NONE	N/A	210 ml	210 ml
5 years Compound	190 ml	NONE	N/A	190 ml	190 ml
4 years Compound	160 ml	NONE	N/A	160 ml	160 ml
3 years Compound	140 ml	NONE	N/A	140 ml	140 ml

*see Medicines: Best Practice checklist **MEDS**

Sodium Lactate Compound   SLC

Burns (10 ml/kg, given over 1 hour) – *continued*:

- TBSA: between 10% and 20% and time to hospital is greater than 30 minutes.
- TBSA: more than 20%.

AGE	INITIAL DOSE	REPEAT DOSE	DOSE INTERVAL	VOLUME	MAXIMUM DOSE
2 years Compound	120 ml	NONE	N/A	120 ml	120 ml
18 months Compound	110 ml	NONE	N/A	110 ml	110 ml
12 months Compound	100 ml	NONE	N/A	100 ml	100 ml
9 months Compound	90 ml	NONE	N/A	90 ml	90 ml
6 months Compound	80 ml	NONE	N/A	80 ml	80 ml
3 months Compound	60 ml	NONE	N/A	60 ml	60 ml
1 month Compound	45 ml	NONE	N/A	45 ml	45 ml
Birth N/A	N/A	N/A	N/A	N/A	N/A

Syntometrine

SYN

Presentation
An ampoule containing ergometrine 500 micrograms and oxytocin 5 units in 1 ml.

Indications
Post-partum haemorrhage within 24 hours of delivery of the infant where bleeding from the uterus is uncontrollable by uterine massage.

Miscarriage with life-threatening bleeding and a confirmed diagnosis (e.g. where a patient has gone home with medical management and starts to bleed).

Actions
Stimulates contraction of the uterus.

Onset of action 7–10 minutes.

Contra-indications
- Known hypersensitivity to syntometrine.
- In labour, prior to the birth of the baby.
- Severe cardiac, liver or kidney disease.
- Hypertension and severe pre-eclampsia.
- Possible multiple pregnancy/known or suspected fetus in utero.

see Medicines: Best Practice checklist · **MEDS**

Syntometrine · SYN

Side Effects

- Nausea and vomiting.
- Abdominal pain.
- Headache.
- Hypertension and bradycardia.
- Chest pain and, rarely, anaphylactic reactions.

Additional Information

Syntometrine and misoprostol reduce bleeding from a pregnant uterus through different pathways; therefore if one drug has not been effective after 15 minutes, the other may be administered in addition.

Dosage and Administration

Route: Intramuscular.

AGE	INITIAL DOSE	REPEAT DOSE	DOSE INTERVAL	VOLUME	MAX DOSE
Adult 500 micrograms of ergometrine and 5 units of oxytocin in 1 ml	500 micrograms of ergometrine and 5 units of oxytocin	None	N/A	1 ml	500 micrograms of ergometrine and 5 units of oxytocin

Tenecteplase   TNK

Presentation

Vials of **tenecteplase** 10,000 units for reconstitution with 10 ml water for injection, or 8,000 units for reconstitution with 8 ml water for injection.

NOTE: Whilst the strength of thrombolytics is traditionally expressed in 'units' these units are unique to each particular drug and are **NOT** interchangeable.

Indications

Acute ST segment elevation MI (STEMI) within 6 hours of symptom onset where primary percutaneous coronary intervention (PPCI) is **NOT** readily available.

Ensure patient fulfils the criteria for drug administration following the model checklist (below). Variation of these criteria is justifiable at local level with agreement of appropriate key stakeholders (e.g. cardiac network, or in the context of an approved clinical trial).

Contra-Indications

Refer to local Trust checklist for thrombolytics.

Actions

Activates the fibrinolytic system, inducing the breaking up of intravascular thrombi and emboli.

see Medicines: Best Practice checklist **MEDS**

Tenecteplase **TNK**

Side Effects

Bleeding:

- Major – seek medical advice and transport to hospital rapidly.
- Minor (e.g. at injection sites) – use local pressure.

Arrhythmias – these are usually benign in the form of transient idioventricular rhythms and usually require no special treatment. Treat ventricular fibrillation (VF) as a complication of myocardial infarction (MI) with standard protocols; bradycardia with atropine as required.

Anaphylaxis – extremely rare (0.1%) with third generation bolus agents.

Hypotension – often responds to laying the patient flat.

Additional Information

PPCI is now the dominant reperfusion treatment and should be used where available; patients with STEMI will be taken direct to a specialist cardiac centre instead of receiving thrombolysis (**refer to Acute Coronary Syndrome**). Local guidelines should be followed.

'Time is muscle!' Do not delay transportation to hospital if difficulties arise whilst setting up the equipment or establishing IV access. Qualified single responders should administer a thrombolytic if indicated while awaiting arrival of an ambulance.

Tenecteplase TNK

In All Cases
Ensure a defibrillator is immediately available at all times.

Monitor conscious level, pulse, blood pressure and cardiac rhythm during and following injections. Manage complications (associated with the acute MI) as they occur using standard protocols. The main early adverse event associated with thrombolysis is bleeding, which should be managed according to standard guidelines.

AT HOSPITAL – emphasise the need to commence a heparin infusion in accordance with local guidelines – to reduce the risk of re-infarction.

Thrombolysis Checklist
Is primary PCI available?
- **YES** – undertake a **TIME CRITICAL** transfer to PPCI capable hospital.
- **NO** – refer to local Trust checklists for thrombolytics.

*see Medicines: Best Practice checklist   **MEDS**

Tenecteplase   **TNK**

Dosage and Administration

1. Administer a bolus of intravenous injection of un-fractionated heparin before administration of tenecteplase (**refer to Heparin**). Flush the cannula well with saline.

2. **AT HOSPITAL** – It is essential that the care of the patient is handed over as soon as possible to a member of hospital staff qualified to administer a heparin infusion.

3. Consider halving the dose in patients aged 75 or over to reduce the risk of intracranial haemorrhage. This will be determined by local pathways.

Route: Intravenous single bolus adjusted for patient weight.

AGE	WEIGHT	INITIAL DOSE	REPEAT DOSE	DOSE INTERVAL	VOLUME	MAXIMUM DOSE
≥**18** 1,000 U/ml	<60 kg (<9st 6lbs)	6,000 units	NONE	N/A	6 ml	6,000 units
≥**18** 1,000 U/ml	60–69 kg (9st 6lbs–10st 13lbs)	7,000 units	NONE	N/A	7 ml	7,000 units
≥**18** 1,000 U/ml	70–79 kg (11st–12st 7lbs)	8,000 units	NONE	N/A	8 ml	8,000 units
≥**18** 1,000 U/ml	80–90 kg (12st 8lbs–14st 2lbs)	9,000 units	NONE	N/A	9 ml	9,000 units
≥**18** 1,000 U/ml	>90 kg (>14st 2lbs)	10,000 units	NONE	N/A	10 ml	10,000 units

Tranexamic Acid TXA

Presentation
Vial containing 500 mg tranexamic acid in 5 ml (100 mg/ml).

Indications
Patients with signs of actual or suspected severe haemorrhage in the following clinical scenarios:

- Injured patients triggering local network major trauma criteria.
- Head injury patients, aged 18 and over with a GCS of 12 or less.
- Patients with a time critical injury where significant internal or external haemorrhage is known or suspected.
- Post-partum haemorrhage if after administration of an uterotonic drug the patient continues to bleed.
- Bleeding due to disorders of obstetric origin.

Trauma

Treatment of known or suspected severe traumatic internal or external haemorrhage as soon as clinically possible on arrival at the scene and within 3 hours of bleeding starting in adults and children who are considered to be at risk of significant haemorrhage. This may be demonstrated by one or more of:

- Systolic blood pressure < 90mmHg or absent radial pulse or heart rate > 110 bpm believed to be due to bleeding in adults. In children this may be demonstrated by changes in the normal physiological parameters for age (see JRCALC page for age).

see Medicines: Best Practice checklist **MEDS**

Tranexamic Acid   **TXA**

- Any patient where haemostatic gauze, arterial tourniquet/s, chest dressing/s or pressure dressing/s have been applied.
- Patient who has suffered a traumatic cardiac arrest.

The above would include women who have recently given birth but have suffered subsequent trauma.

Women who are pregnant and/or breastfeeding should have tranexamic acid administered in life threatening circumstances.

Head Injury

Patients aged 18 and over who have a known or suspected head injury where the following criteria is met:

- The GCS is 12 or less.
- The injury has occurred within the last 3 hours.

Post-Partum Haemorrhage

Either of the following criteria:

- Woman who has given birth within 3 hours, with post-partum haemorrhage causing haemodynamic instability (has lost 500ml or more of blood) **which has not responded to the administration of an uterotonic drug**.
- Woman with a post-partum haemorrhage when uterine trauma (rupture) is suspected.
- Woman for whom uterotonic drugs are contraindicated (i.e. patient has high blood pressure).
- Women who are breastfeeding should have tranexamic acid administered in life threatening circumstances.

Tranexamic Acid TXA

Obstetric Emergencies

Life-threatening bleeding due to disorders of obstetric origin.

Women who are pregnant and/or breastfeeding should have tranexamic acid administered in life threatening circumstances.

Actions

Tranexamic acid is an anti-fibrinolytic which reduces the breakdown of a blood clot.

Contra-Indications

- Known previous anaphylactic reaction to Tranexamic Acid.
- Bleeding started more than 3 hours ago.
- Obvious resolution of haemorrhage.
- Post-partum haemorrhage before the administration of an uterotonic unless trauma is suspected cause.
- Critical interventions required (must only be given after critical interventions have been performed: i.e. airway managed; control or splinting of major haemorrhage etc. and if administration does not delay transfer, noting it may be administered en route).

Cautions

Contact the local senior on call clinician for advice on the below if required:

- Patients with a known history of convulsions or convulsions from any cause during the incident. High dose regimes have been associated

*see Medicines: Best Practice checklist **MEDS**

Tranexamic Acid   TXA

with convulsions; however, in the low dose regime recommended here, the benefit from giving tranexamic acid for severe haemorrhage outweighs the risk of convulsions. An increase in convulsion rate may be due to the antagonistic effect of tranexamic acid on GABA receptors. Treat convulsions which may be caused by treatment with tranexamic acid as per JRCALC and Trust guidance (management not covered under this PGD).

- Patients with a known history of acute venous or arterial thrombosis. In the low dose regime recommended here, the benefit from giving tranexamic acid for severe haemorrhage outweighs the risk of thrombotic events. This information should be passed to the receiving hospital.

- Patients with known severe renal impairment (eGFR <30 ml/min 1.73 m^2). There is a risk of accumulation of tranexamic acid. In the low dose regime recommended here, the benefit from giving tranexamic acid for severe haemorrhage outweighs the risk of accumulation. This information should be passed to the receiving hospital.

- Rapid injection may cause hypotension and loss of consciousness.

- Do not administer through the same line as blood products or penicillin antibiotics (including co-amoxiclav).

Side Effects

Common side effects (more than 1 in 100 but less than 1 in 10)

- Nausea.

- Vomiting.

- Diarrhoea.

Tranexamic Acid — TXA

Serious adverse effects (unknown rate of incidence)

- Hypersensitivity reactions including anaphylaxis have been reported.
- Rapid injection may cause hypotension.
- Arterial or venous embolism at any site.

Dosage and Administration

Route: Intravenous/Intraosseous – **administer SLOWLY over 10 minutes – can be given as 10 aliquots administered 1 minute apart.**

Post-partum haemorrhage in women: A second dose can be administered if bleeding continues after 30 minutes of the first dose being administered. Any further doses are not permissible within 24 hours.

AGE	INITIAL DOSE	REPEAT DOSE	DOSE INTERVAL	VOLUME	MAX DOSE
>12 years – Adult 100 mg/ml	1 gram	NONE	N/A	10 ml	1 gram

PAGE FOR AGE

Page for Age

BIRTH*

Vital Signs

GUIDE WEIGHT	HEART RATE	RESPIRATION RATE	SYSTOLIC BLOOD PRESSURE
3.5 kg	110–160	30–40	70–90

Airway Size by Type

OROPHARYNGEAL AIRWAY	LARYNGEAL MASK	I-GEL AIRWAY	ENDOTRACHEAL TUBE
000	1	1	Diameter: **3 mm**; Length: **10 cm**

Intravascular Fluid

FLUID	INITIAL DOSE	REPEAT DOSE	DOSE INTERVAL	VOLUME	MAX DOSE
Sodium Chloride (5 ml/kg) (IV/IO) 0.9%	20 ml	20 ml	PRN	20 ml	140 ml
Sodium Chloride (10ml/kg) (IV/IO) 0.9%	35 ml	35 ml	PRN	35 ml	140 ml
Sodium Chloride (20 ml/kg) (IV/IO) 0.9%	70 ml	70 ml	PRN	70 ml	140 ml

*The Page for Age is provided for ease of use and quick look purposes. It is not a substitute for the information contained in the complete drugs guidelines or for sound clinical judgement.

PAGE AGE

Cardiac Arrest — Page for Age

BIRTH

DRUG	INITIAL DOSE	REPEAT DOSE	DOSE INTERVAL	VOLUME	MAX DOSE
ADRENALINE **Cardiac Arrest** (IV/IO) 1 milligram in 10 ml (1:10,000)	35 micrograms	35 micrograms	3–5 minutes	**0.35 ml**	No limit

Quick Reference Table — BIRTH — Page for Age

DRUG	INITIAL DOSE	REPEAT DOSE	DOSE INTERVAL	VOLUME	MAX DOSE
ACTIVATED CHARCOAL (Oral)	N/A	N/A	N/A	N/A	N/A
ADRENALINE - ANAPHYLAXIS/ASTHMA (IM) 1 milligram in 1 ml (1:1,000)	150 micrograms	150 micrograms	5 minutes	0.15 ml	No limit
BENZYLPENICILLIN (IV/IO) 600 milligrams dissolved in 10 ml water for injection	300 milligrams	NONE	N/A	5 ml	300 milligrams
BENZYLPENICILLIN (IM) 600 milligrams dissolved in 2 ml water for injection	300 milligrams	NONE	N/A	1 ml	300 milligrams
CHLORPHENAMINE (IV/IO/IM)	N/A	N/A	N/A	N/A	N/A
CHLORPHENAMINE Oral (tablet)	N/A	N/A	N/A	N/A	N/A
CHLORPHENAMINE Oral (solution)	N/A	N/A	N/A	N/A	N/A
DEXAMETHASONE (Oral)	N/A	N/A	N/A	N/A	N/A

Quick Reference Table

BIRTH
Page for Age

DRUG	INITIAL DOSE	REPEAT DOSE	DOSE INTERVAL	VOLUME	MAX DOSE
DIAZEPAM (IV/IO) 10 milligrams in 2 ml	1 milligram	1 milligram	10 minutes	0.2 ml	2 milligrams
DIAZEPAM (Rectal) 2.5 milligrams in 1.25 ml	1.25 milligrams	1.25 milligrams	10 minutes	0.5 x 2.5 milligram tube	2.5 milligram
GLUCAGON (IM) 1 milligram per vial	100 micrograms	NONE	N/A	0.1 vial	100 micrograms
GLUCOSE 10% (IV) 50 grams in 500 ml	900 milligrams	900 milligrams	5 minutes	9 ml	27 ml (2.7 g glucose)
GLUCOSE 40% ORAL GEL (Buccal) 10 grams in 25 grams of gel	An appropriate amount should be administered, considering the child's size	See initial dose	5 minutes	1 tube	An appropriate amount should be administered, considering the child's size
HYDROCORTISONE (IV/IO/IM) 100 milligrams in 1 ml	10 milligrams	NONE	N/A	0.1 ml	10 milligrams
HYDROCORTISONE (IV/IO/IM) 100 milligrams	10 milligrams	NONE	N/A	0.2 ml	10 milligrams
IBUPROFEN (Oral) in 2 ml	N/A	N/A	N/A	N/A	N/A

Quick Reference Table — BIRTH — Page for Age

DRUG	INITIAL DOSE	REPEAT DOSE	DOSE INTERVAL	VOLUME	MAX DOSE
IPRATROPIUM BROMIDE (Neb)	N/A	N/A	N/A	N/A	N/A
IPRATROPIUM BROMIDE (Neb)	N/A	N/A	N/A	N/A	N/A
MIDAZOLAM* (Buccal) 5 milligrams in 1 ml	See Epilepsy Passport	See Epilepsy Passport	10 mins	See Epilepsy Passport	See Epilepsy Passport
MORPHINE SULFATE (IV/IO)	N/A	N/A	N/A	N/A	N/A
MORPHINE SULFATE (Oral)	N/A	N/A	N/A	N/A	N/A
NALOXONE (IV/IO)	N/A	N/A	N/A	N/A	N/A
NALOXONE (IM)	N/A	N/A	N/A	N/A	N/A
ONDANSETRON (IV/IO/IM)	N/A	N/A	N/A	N/A	N/A
PARACETAMOL - INFANT SUSPENSION (Oral)	N/A	N/A	N/A	N/A	N/A

*Give the dose as prescribed in the child's individual treatment plan/Epilepsy Passport (the dosages described above reflect the recommended dosages for a child of this age).

PAGE AGE

Quick Reference Table

BIRTH — Page for Age

DRUG	INITIAL DOSE	REPEAT DOSE	DOSE INTERVAL	VOLUME	MAX DOSE
PARACETAMOL (IV infusion/IO) 10 milligrams in 1 ml	35 milligrams	35 milligrams	4–6 hours	3.5ml	105 milligrams in 24 hours
SALBUTAMOL (Neb)	N/A	N/A	N/A	N/A	N/A
SALBUTAMOL (Neb)	N/A	N/A	N/A	N/A	N/A
TRANEXAMIC ACID (IV) 100 mg/ml	50 mg	NONE	N/A	**0.5 ml**	50 mg

251

Page for Age

1 MONTH

Vital Signs

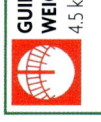

GUIDE WEIGHT	HEART RATE	RESPIRATION RATE	SYSTOLIC BLOOD PRESSURE
4.5 kg	110–160	30–40	70–90

Airway Size by Type

OROPHARYNGEAL AIRWAY	LARYNGEAL MASK	I-GEL AIRWAY	ENDOTRACHEAL TUBE
00	1	1	Diameter: **3 mm**; Length: **10 cm**

Defibrillation – Cardiac Arrest

MANUAL	AUTOMATED EXTERNAL DEFIBRILLATOR
20 Joules	Where possible, use a manual defibrillator. If an AED is the only defibrillator available, it should be used (preferably using paediatric attenuation pads or else in paediatric mode).

Intravascular Fluid

FLUID	INITIAL DOSE	REPEAT DOSE	DOSE INTERVAL	VOLUME	MAX DOSE
Sodium Chloride (5 ml/kg) 0.9% (IV/IO)	20 ml	20 ml	PRN	20 ml	180 ml
Sodium Chloride (10 ml/kg) 0.9% (IV/IO)	45 ml	45 ml	PRN	45 ml	180 ml
Sodium Chloride (20 ml/kg) 0.9% (IV/IO)	90 ml	90 ml	PRN	90 ml	180 ml

Cardiac Arrest

1 MONTH — Page for Age

DRUG	INITIAL DOSE	REPEAT DOSE	DOSE INTERVAL	VOLUME	MAX DOSE
ADRENALINE **Cardiac Arrest** (IV/IO) 1 milligram in 10 ml (1:10,000)	50 micrograms	50 micrograms	3–5 minutes	0.5 ml	No limit
AMIODARONE **Cardiac Arrest** (IV/IO) 300 milligrams in 10 ml	25 milligrams (After 3rd shock)	25 milligrams	After 5th shock	0.8 ml	50 milligrams

Quick Reference Table — 1 MONTH — Page for Age

DRUG	INITIAL DOSE	REPEAT DOSE	DOSE INTERVAL	VOLUME	MAX DOSE
ACTIVATED CHARCOAL (Oral)	N/A	N/A	N/A	N/A	N/A
ADRENALINE - ANAPHYLAXIS/ASTHMA (IM) 1 milligram in 1 ml (1:1,000)	150 micrograms	150 micrograms	5 minutes	0.15 ml	No limit
BENZYLPENICILLIN (IV/IO) 600 milligrams dissolved in 10 ml water for injection	300 milligrams	NONE	N/A	5 ml	300 milligrams
BENZYLPENICILLIN (IM) 600 milligrams dissolved in 2 ml water for injection	300 milligrams	NONE	N/A	1 ml	300 milligrams
CHLORPHENAMINE (IV/IO/IM) 10 milligrams in 1 ml	1 milligram	NONE	N/A	0.1 ml	1 milligram
CHLORPHENAMINE Oral (tablet)	N/A	N/A	N/A	N/A	N/A
CHLORPHENAMINE Oral (solution) 2 milligrams in 5 ml	1 milligram	NONE	N/A	2.5 ml	1 milligram

Quick Reference Table

1 MONTH — Page for Age

DRUG	INITIAL DOSE	REPEAT DOSE	DOSE INTERVAL	VOLUME	MAX DOSE
DEXAMETHASONE Oral (solution) 2 milligrams in 5 ml	0.8 milligram	NONE	N/A	2 ml	0.8 milligram
DEXAMETHASONE Oral (tablet) 2 milligrams per tablet	2 milligrams	NONE	N/A	1 tablet	2 milligrams
DIAZEPAM (IV/IO) 10 milligrams in 2 ml	1.5 milligrams	1.5 milligrams	10 minutes	0.3 ml	3 milligrams
DIAZEPAM (Rectal) 2.5 milligrams in 1.25 ml	2.5 milligrams	2.5 milligrams	10 minutes	1 x 2.5 milligram tube	5 milligrams
GLUCAGON (IM) 1 milligram per vial	500 micrograms	NONE	N/A	0.5 vial	500 micrograms
GLUCOSE 10% (IV) 50 grams in 500 ml	1 gram glucose	1 gram glucose	5 minutes	10 ml	30 ml (3 g glucose)
GLUCOSE 40% ORAL GEL (Buccal) 10 grams in 25 grams of gel	An appropriate amount should be administered, considering the child's size	See initial dose	5 minutes	1 tube	An appropriate amount should be administered, considering the child's size

255

Quick Reference Table — 1 MONTH — Page for Age

DRUG	INITIAL DOSE	REPEAT DOSE	DOSE INTERVAL	VOLUME	MAX DOSE
HYDROCORTISONE (IV/IO/IM) 100 milligrams in 1 ml	25 milligrams	NONE	N/A	0.25 ml	25 milligrams
HYDROCORTISONE (IV/IO/IM) 100 milligrams in 2 ml	25 milligrams	NONE	N/A	0.5 ml	25 milligrams
IBUPROFEN (Oral)	N/A	N/A	N/A	N/A	N/A
IPRATROPIUM BROMIDE (Neb) 500 micrograms in 2 ml	125–250 micrograms	NONE	N/A	0.5 ml–1 ml	125–250 micrograms
IPRATROPIUM BROMIDE (Neb) 250 micrograms in 1 ml	125–250 micrograms	NONE	N/A	0.5 ml–1 ml	125–250 micrograms
MIDAZOLAM* (Buccal) 5 milligrams in 1 ml	See Epilepsy Passport	See Epilepsy Passport	10 mins	See Epilepsy Passport	See Epilepsy Passport
MORPHINE SULFATE (IV/IO)	N/A	N/A	N/A	N/A	N/A

*Give the dose as prescribed in the child's individual treatment plan/Epilepsy Passport (the dosages described above reflect the recommended dosages for a child of this age).

Quick Reference Table

1 MONTH — Page for Age

DRUG	INITIAL DOSE	REPEAT DOSE	DOSE INTERVAL	VOLUME	MAX DOSE
MORPHINE SULFATE (Oral)	N/A	N/A	N/A	N/A	N/A
NALOXONE (IV/IO) 400 micrograms in 1 ml	400 micrograms	400 micrograms	1 minute	1 ml	2,000 micrograms
NALOXONE (IM) 400 micrograms in 1 ml	400 micrograms	400 micrograms	3 minutes	1 ml	2,000 micrograms
ONDANSETRON (IV/IO/IM) 2 milligrams in 1 ml	0.5 milligrams	NONE	N/A	0.25 ml	0.5 milligrams
PARACETAMOL - INFANT SUSPENSION (Oral)	N/A	N/A	N/A	N/A	N/A
PARACETAMOL IV infusion/IO 10 milligrams in 1 ml	45 milligrams	45 milligrams	4-6 hours	4.5 ml	135 milligrams in 24 hours
SALBUTAMOL (Neb) 2.5 milligrams in 2.5 ml	2.5 milligrams	2.5 milligrams	5 minutes	2.5 ml	No limit

Quick Reference Table   **1 MONTH**   Page for Age

DRUG	INITIAL DOSE	REPEAT DOSE	DOSE INTERVAL	VOLUME	MAX DOSE
SALBUTAMOL (Neb) 5 milligrams in 2.5 ml	2.5 milligrams	2.5 milligrams	5 minutes	1.25 ml	No limit
TRANEXAMIC ACID (IV) 100 mg/ml	50 mg	NONE	N/A	0.5 ml	50 mg

This page left intentionally blank for your notes

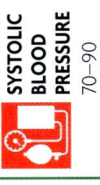

Page for Age

3 MONTHS

Vital Signs

GUIDE WEIGHT	HEART RATE	RESPIRATION RATE	SYSTOLIC BLOOD PRESSURE
6 kg	110–160	30–40	70–90

Airway Size by Type

OROPHARYNGEAL AIRWAY	LARYNGEAL MASK	I-GEL AIRWAY	ENDOTRACHEAL TUBE
00	1.5	1.5	Diameter: **3.5 mm**; Length: **11 cm**

Defibrillation – Cardiac Arrest

MANUAL	AUTOMATED EXTERNAL DEFIBRILLATOR
25 Joules	Where possible, use a manual defibrillator. If an AED is the only defibrillator available, it should be used (preferably using paediatric attenuation pads or else in paediatric mode).

Intravascular Fluid

FLUID	INITIAL DOSE	REPEAT DOSE	DOSE INTERVAL	VOLUME	MAX DOSE
Sodium Chloride (5 ml/kg) (IV/IO) 0.9%	30 ml	30 ml	PRN	30 ml	240 ml
Sodium Chloride (10 ml/kg) (IV/IO) 0.9%	60 ml	60 ml	PRN	60 ml	240 ml
Sodium Chloride (20 ml/kg) (IV/IO) 0.9%	120 ml	120 ml	PRN	120 ml	240 ml

3 MONTHS Page for Age

DRUG	INITIAL DOSE	REPEAT DOSE	DOSE INTERVAL	VOLUME	MAX DOSE
ADRENALINE Cardiac Arrest (IV/IO) 1 milligram in 10 ml (1:10,000)	60 micrograms	60 micrograms	3–5 minutes	0.6 ml	No limit
AMIODARONE Cardiac Arrest (IV/IO) 300 milligrams in 10 ml	30 milligrams (After 3rd shock)	30 milligrams	After 5th shock	1 ml	60 milligrams

Quick Reference Table — 3 MONTHS Page for Age

DRUG	INITIAL DOSE	REPEAT DOSE	DOSE INTERVAL	VOLUME	MAX DOSE
ACTIVATED CHARCOAL (Oral)	N/A	N/A	N/A	N/A	N/A
ADRENALINE - ANAPHYLAXIS/ ASTHMA (IM) 1 milligram in 1 ml (1:1,000)	150 micrograms	150 micrograms	5 minutes	0.15 ml	No limit
BENZYLPENICILLIN (IV/IO) 600 milligrams dissolved in 10 ml water for injection	300 milligrams	NONE	N/A	5 ml	300 milligrams
BENZYLPENICILLIN (IM) 600 milligrams dissolved in 2 ml water for injection	300 milligrams	NONE	N/A	1 ml	300 milligrams
CHLORPHENAMINE (IV/IO/IM) 10 milligrams in 1 ml	1 milligram	NONE	N/A	0.1 ml	1 milligram
CHLORPHENAMINE Oral (tablet)	N/A	N/A	N/A	N/A	N/A
CHLORPHENAMINE Oral (solution) 2 milligrams in 5 ml	1 milligram	NONE	N/A	2.5 ml	1 milligram

Quick Reference Table

3 MONTHS Page for Age

DRUG	INITIAL DOSE	REPEAT DOSE	DOSE INTERVAL	VOLUME	MAX DOSE
DEXAMETHASONE Oral (solution) 2 milligrams in 5 ml	1.2 milligram	NONE	N/A	3 ml	1.2 milligram
DEXAMETHASONE Oral (tablet) 2 milligrams per tablet	2 milligrams	NONE	N/A	1 tablet	2 milligrams
DIAZEPAM (IV/IO) 10 milligrams in 2 ml	2 milligrams	2 milligrams	10 minutes	0.4 ml	4 milligrams
DIAZEPAM (Rectal) 2.5 milligrams in 1.25 ml	2.5 milligrams	2.5 milligrams	10 minutes	1 x 2.5 milligram tube	5 milligrams
GLUCAGON (IM) 1 milligram per vial	500 micrograms	NONE	N/A	0.5 vial	500 micrograms
GLUCOSE 10% (IV) 50 grams in 500 ml	1 gram glucose	1 gram glucose	5 minutes	10 ml	30 ml (3 g glucose)
GLUCOSE 40% ORAL GEL Buccal) 10 grams in 25 grams of gel	An appropriate amount should be administered, considering the child's size	See initial dose	5 minutes	1 tube	An appropriate amount should be administered, considering the child's size
HYDROCORTISONE (IV/IO /IM) 100 milligrams in 1 ml	25 milligrams	NONE	N/A	0.25 ml	25 milligrams

263

Quick Reference Table — 3 MONTHS — Page for Age

DRUG	INITIAL DOSE	REPEAT DOSE	DOSE INTERVAL	VOLUME	MAX DOSE
HYDROCORTISONE (IV/IO/IM) 100 milligrams in 2 ml	25 milligrams	NONE	N/A	0.5 ml	25 milligrams
IBUPROFEN (Oral) 100 milligrams in 5 ml	50 milligrams	50 milligrams	8 hours	2.5 ml	150 milligrams per 24 hours
IPRATROPIUM BROMIDE (Neb) 250 micrograms in 1 ml	125–250 micrograms	NONE	N/A	0.5 ml–1 ml	125–250 micrograms
IPRATROPIUM BROMIDE (Neb) 500 micrograms in 2 ml	125–250 micrograms	NONE	N/A	0.5 ml–1 ml	125–250 micrograms
MIDAZOLAM* (Buccal) 5 milligrams in 1 ml	See Epilepsy Passport	See Epilepsy Passport	10 mins	See Epilepsy Passport	See Epilepsy Passport
MORPHINE SULFATE (IV/IO)	N/A	N/A	N/A	N/A	N/A
MORPHINE SULFATE (Oral)	N/A	N/A	N/A	N/A	N/A

*Give the dose as prescribed in the child's individual treatment plan/Epilepsy Passport (the dosages described above reflect the recommended dosages for a child of this age).

Quick Reference Table — 3 MONTHS Page for Age

DRUG	INITIAL DOSE	REPEAT DOSE	DOSE INTERVAL	VOLUME	MAX DOSE
NALOXONE (IM) 400 micrograms in 1 ml	400 micrograms	400 micrograms	1 minute	1 ml	2,000 micrograms
NALOXONE (IV/IO/IM) 400 micrograms in 1 ml	400 micrograms	400 micrograms	3 minutes	1 ml	2,000 micrograms
ONDANSETRON (IV/IO/IM) 2 milligrams in 1 ml	0.5 milligrams	NONE	N/A	0.25 ml	0.5 milligrams
PARACETAMOL - INFANT SUSPENSION (Oral) 120 milligrams in 5 ml	60 milligrams	60 milligrams	4–6 hours	2.5 ml	240 milligrams in 24 hours
PARACETAMOL (IV infusion/IO) 10 milligrams in 1 ml	60 milligrams	60 milligrams	4–6 hours	6 ml	180 milligrams in 24 hours
SALBUTAMOL (Neb) 2.5 milligrams in 2.5 ml	2.5 milligrams	2.5 milligrams	5 minutes	2.5 ml	No limit
SALBUTAMOL (Neb) 5 milligrams in 2.5 ml	2.5 milligrams	2.5 milligrams	5 minutes	1.25 ml	No limit
TRANEXAMIC ACID (IV) 100 mg/ml	100 mg	NONE	N/A	1 ml	100 mg

265

Page for Age

6 MONTHS

Vital Signs

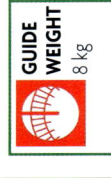

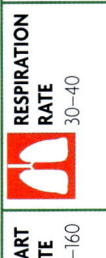

GUIDE WEIGHT	HEART RATE	RESPIRATION RATE	SYSTOLIC BLOOD PRESSURE
8 kg	110–160	30–40	70–90

Airway Size by Type

OROPHARYNGEAL AIRWAY	LARYNGEAL MASK	I-GEL AIRWAY	ENDOTRACHEAL TUBE
00	1.5	1.5	Diameter: **4 mm**; Length: **12 cm**

Defibrillation – Cardiac Arrest

MANUAL	AUTOMATED EXTERNAL DEFIBRILLATOR
40 Joules	Where possible, use a manual defibrillator. If an AED is the only defibrillator available, it should be used (preferably using paediatric attenuation pads or else in paediatric mode).

Intravascular Fluid

FLUID	INITIAL DOSE	REPEAT DOSE	DOSE INTERVAL	VOLUME	MAX DOSE
Sodium Chloride (5 ml/kg) (IV/IO) 0.9%	40 ml	40 ml	PRN	40 ml	320 ml
Sodium Chloride (10 ml/kg) (IV/IO) 0.9%	80 ml	80 ml	PRN	80 ml	320 ml
Sodium Chloride (20 ml/kg) (IV/IO) 0.9%	160 ml	160 ml	PRN	160 ml	320 ml

6 MONTHS Page for Age

Cardiac Arrest

DRUG	INITIAL DOSE	REPEAT DOSE	DOSE INTERVAL	VOLUME	MAX DOSE
ADRENALINE **Cardiac Arrest** (IV/O) 1 milligram in 10 ml (1:10,000)	80 micrograms	80 micrograms	3–5 minutes	0.8 ml	No limit
AMIODARONE **Cardiac Arrest** (IV/O) 300 milligrams in 10 ml	40 milligrams (After 3rd shock)	40 milligrams	After 5th shock	1.3 ml	80 milligrams

267

Quick Reference Table — 6 MONTHS — Page for Age

DRUG	INITIAL DOSE	REPEAT DOSE	DOSE INTERVAL	VOLUME	MAX DOSE
ACTIVATED CHARCOAL (Oral)	N/A	N/A	N/A	N/A	N/A
ADRENALINE - ANAPHYLAXIS/ASTHMA (IM) 1 milligram in 1 ml (1:1,000)	150 micrograms	150 micrograms	5 minutes	0.15 ml	No limit
BENZYLPENICILLIN (IV/IO) 600 milligrams dissolved in 10 ml water for injection	300 milligrams	NONE	N/A	5 ml	300 milligrams
BENZYLPENICILLIN (IM) 600 milligrams dissolved in 2 ml water for injection	300 milligrams	NONE	N/A	1 ml	300 milligrams
CHLORPHENAMINE (IV/IO/IM) 10 milligrams in 1 ml	2.5 milligrams	NONE	N/A	0.25 ml	2.5 milligrams
CHLORPHENAMINE Oral (tablet)	N/A	N/A	N/A	N/A	N/A
CHLORPHENAMINE Oral (solution) 2 milligrams in 5 ml	1 milligram	NONE	N/A	2.5 ml	1 milligram

Quick Reference Table

6 MONTHS Page for Age

DRUG	INITIAL DOSE	REPEAT DOSE	DOSE INTERVAL	VOLUME	MAX DOSE
DEXAMETHASONE Oral (solution) 2 milligrams in 5 ml	1.6 milligram	NONE	N/A	4 ml	1.6 milligram
DEXAMETHASONE Oral (tablet) 2 milligrams per tablet	2 milligrams	NONE	N/A	1 tablet	2 milligrams
DIAZEPAM (IV/IO) 10 milligrams in 2 ml	2.5 milligrams	2.5 milligrams	10 minutes	0.5 ml	5 milligrams
DIAZEPAM (Rectal) 5 milligrams in 2.5 ml	5 milligrams	5 milligrams	10 minutes	1 x 5 milligram tube	10 milligrams
GLUCAGON (IM) 1 milligram per vial	500 micrograms	NONE	N/A	0.5 vial	500 micrograms
GLUCOSE 10% (IV) 50 grams in 500 ml	1.5 grams glucose	1.5 grams glucose	5 minutes	15 ml	45 ml (4.5 g glucose)
GLUCOSE 40% ORAL GEL (Buccal) 10 grams in 25 grams of gel	An appropriate amount should be administered, considering the child's size	See initial dose	5 minutes	1 tube	An appropriate amount should be administered, considering the child's size
HYDROCORTISONE (IV/IO/IM) 100 milligrams in 1 ml	50 milligrams	NONE	N/A	0.5 ml	50 milligrams

269

Quick Reference Table — 6 MONTHS — Page for Age

DRUG	INITIAL DOSE	REPEAT DOSE	DOSE INTERVAL	VOLUME	MAX DOSE
HYDROCORTISONE (IV/IO/IM) 100 milligrams in 2 ml	50 milligrams	NONE	N/A	1 ml	50 milligrams
IBUPROFEN (Oral) 100 milligrams in 5 ml	50 milligrams	50 milligrams	8 hours	2.5 ml	150 milligrams per 24 hours
IPRATROPIUM BROMIDE (Neb) 250 micrograms in 1 ml	125–250 micrograms	NONE	N/A	0.5 ml–1 ml	125–250 micrograms
IPRATROPIUM BROMIDE (Neb) 500 micrograms in 2 ml	125–250 micrograms	NONE	N/A	0.5 ml–1 ml	125–250 micrograms
MIDAZOLAM* (Buccal) 5 milligrams in 1 ml	2.5 milligrams	2.5 milligrams	10 mins	0.5 ml pre-filled syringe	5 milligrams
MORPHINE SULFATE (IV/IO)	N/A	N/A	N/A	N/A	N/A
MORPHINE SULFATE (Oral)	N/A	N/A	N/A	N/A	N/A

*Give the dose as prescribed in the child's individual treatment plan/Epilepsy Passport (the dosages described above reflect the recommended dosages for a child of this age).

Quick Reference Table

6 MONTHS Page for Age

DRUG	INITIAL DOSE	REPEAT DOSE	DOSE INTERVAL	VOLUME	MAX DOSE
NALOXONE (IV/IO) 400 micrograms in 1 ml	800 micrograms	800 micrograms then 400 micrograms	1 minute	2 ml	2,000 micrograms
NALOXONE (IM) 400 micrograms in 1 ml	400 micrograms	400 micrograms	3 minutes	1 ml	2,000 micrograms
ONDANSETRON (IV/IO/IM) 2 milligrams in 1 ml	1 milligram	NONE	N/A	0.5 ml	1 milligram
PARACETAMOL - INFANT SUSPENSION (Oral) 120 milligrams in 5 ml	120 milligrams	120 milligrams	4–6 hours	5 ml	480 milligrams in 24 hours
PARACETAMOL (IV infusion/IO) 10 milligrams in 1 ml	80 milligrams	80 milligrams	4–6 hours	8 ml	240 milligrams in 24 hours
SALBUTAMOL (Neb) 2.5 milligrams in 2.5 ml	2.5 milligrams	2.5 milligrams	5 minutes	2.5 ml	No limit
SALBUTAMOL (Neb) 5 milligrams in 2.5 ml	2.5 milligrams	2.5 milligrams	5 minutes	1.25 ml	No limit
TRANEXAMIC ACID (IV) 100 mg/ml	100 mg	NONE	N/A	1 ml	100 mg

271

9 MONTHS — Page for Age

Vital Signs

GUIDE WEIGHT	HEART RATE	RESPIRATION RATE	SYSTOLIC BLOOD PRESSURE
9 kg	110–160	30–40	70–90

Airway Size by Type

OROPHARYNGEAL AIRWAY	LARYNGEAL MASK	I-GEL AIRWAY	ENDOTRACHEAL TUBE
00	1.5	1.5	Diameter: **4 mm**; Length: **12 cm**

Defibrillation – Cardiac Arrest

MANUAL	AUTOMATED EXTERNAL DEFIBRILLATOR
40 Joules	Where possible, use a manual defibrillator. If an AED is the only defibrillator available, it should be used (preferably using paediatric attenuation pads or else in paediatric mode).

Intravascular Fluid

FLUID	INITIAL DOSE	REPEAT DOSE	DOSE INTERVAL	VOLUME	MAX DOSE
Sodium Chloride (5 ml/kg) (IV/IO) 0.9%	45 ml	45 ml	PRN	45 ml	360 ml
Sodium Chloride (10 ml/kg) (IV/IO) 0.9%	90 ml	90 ml	PRN	90 ml	360 ml
Sodium Chloride (20 ml/kg) (IV/IO) 0.9%	180 ml	180 ml	PRN	180 ml	360 ml

Cardiac Arrest

9 MONTHS Page for Age

DRUG	INITIAL DOSE	REPEAT DOSE	DOSE INTERVAL	VOLUME	MAX DOSE
ADRENALINE Cardiac Arrest (IV/IO) 1 milligram in 10 ml (1:10,000)	90 micrograms	90 micrograms	3–5 minutes	0.9 ml	No limit
AMIODARONE Cardiac Arrest (IV/IO) 300 milligrams in 10 ml	45 milligrams (After 3rd shock)	45 milligrams	After 5th shock	1.5 ml	90 milligrams

Quick Reference Table — 9 MONTHS — Page for Age

DRUG	INITIAL DOSE	REPEAT DOSE	DOSE INTERVAL	VOLUME	MAX DOSE
ACTIVATED CHARCOAL (Oral)	N/A	N/A	N/A	N/A	N/A
ADRENALINE - ANAPHYLAXIS/ASTHMA (IM) 1 milligram in 1 ml (1:1,000)	150 micrograms	150 micrograms	5 minutes	0.15 ml	No limit
BENZYLPENICILLIN (IV/IO) 600 milligrams dissolved in 10 ml water for injection	300 milligrams	NONE	N/A	5 ml	300 milligrams
BENZYLPENICILLIN (IM) 600 milligrams dissolved in 2 ml water for injection	300 milligrams	NONE	N/A	1 ml	300 milligrams
CHLORPHENAMINE (IV/IO/IM) 10 milligrams in 1 ml	2.5 milligrams	NONE	N/A	0.25 ml	2.5 milligrams
CHLORPHENAMINE Oral (tablet)	N/A	N/A	N/A	N/A	N/A
CHLORPHENAMINE Oral (solution) 2 milligrams in 5 ml	1 milligram	NONE	N/A	2.5 ml	1 milligram

Quick Reference Table

9 MONTHS Page for Age

DRUG	INITIAL DOSE	REPEAT DOSE	DOSE INTERVAL	VOLUME	MAX DOSE
DEXAMETHASONE Oral (solution) 2 milligrams in 5 ml	1.6 milligram	NONE	N/A	4 ml	1.6 milligram
DEXAMETHASONE Oral (tablet) 2 milligrams per tablet	2 milligrams	NONE	N/A	1 tablet	2 milligrams
DIAZEPAM (IV/IO) 10 milligrams in 2 ml	3 milligrams	3 milligrams	10 minutes	0.6 ml	6 milligrams
DIAZEPAM (Rectal) 5 milligrams in 2.5 ml	5 milligrams	5 milligrams	10 minutes	1 x 5 milligram tube	10 milligrams
GLUCAGON (IM) 1 milligram per vial	500 micrograms	NONE	N/A	0.5 vial	500 micrograms
GLUCOSE 10% (IV) 50 grams in 500 ml	2 grams glucose	2 grams glucose	5 minutes	20 ml	60 ml (6 g glucose)
GLUCOSE 40% ORAL GEL (Buccal) 10 grams in 25 grams of gel	An appropriate amount should be administered, considering the child's size	See initial dose	5 minutes	1 tube	An appropriate amount should be administered, considering the child's size
HYDROCORTISONE (IV/IO/IM) 100 milligrams in 1 ml	50 milligrams	NONE	N/A	0.5 ml	50 milligrams

Quick Reference Table — 9 MONTHS — Page for Age

DRUG	INITIAL DOSE	REPEAT DOSE	DOSE INTERVAL	VOLUME	MAX DOSE
HYDROCORTISONE (IV/IO/IM) 100 milligrams in 2 ml	50 milligrams	NONE	N/A	1 ml	50 milligrams
IBUPROFEN (Oral) 100 milligrams in 5 ml	50 milligrams	50 milligrams	8 hours	2.5 ml	150 milligrams per 24 hours
IPRATROPIUM BROMIDE (Neb) 250 micrograms in 1 ml	125–250 micrograms	NONE	N/A	0.5 ml–1 ml	125–250 micrograms
IPRATROPIUM BROMIDE (Neb) 500 micrograms in 2 ml	125–250 micrograms	NONE	N/A	0.5 ml–1 ml	125–250 micrograms
MIDAZOLAM* (Buccal) 5 milligrams in 1 ml	2.5 milligrams	2.5 milligrams	10 mins	0.5 ml pre-filled syringe	5 milligrams
MORPHINE SULFATE (IV/IO)	N/A	N/A	N/A	N/A	N/A
MORPHINE SULFATE (Oral)	N/A	N/A	N/A	N/A	N/A
NALOXONE (IV/IO) 400 micrograms in 1 ml	800 micrograms	800 micrograms then 400 micrograms	1 minute	2 ml	2,000 micrograms

*Give the dose as prescribed in the child's individual treatment plan/Epilepsy Passport (the dosages described above reflect the recommended dosages for a child of this age).

Quick Reference Table

9 MONTHS Page for Age

DRUG	INITIAL DOSE	REPEAT DOSE	DOSE INTERVAL	VOLUME	MAX DOSE
NALOXONE (IM) 400 micrograms in 1 ml	400 micrograms	400 micrograms	3 minutes	1 ml	2,000 micrograms
ONDANSETRON (IV/IO/IM) 2 milligrams in 1 ml	1 milligram	NONE	N/A	0.5 ml	1 milligram
PARACETAMOL - INFANT SUSPENSION (Oral) 120 milligrams in 5 ml	120 milligrams	120 milligrams	4–6 hours	5 ml	480 milligrams in 24 hours
PARACETAMOL (IV infusion/IO) 10 milligrams in 1 ml	90 milligrams	90 milligrams	4–6 hours	9 ml	270 milligrams in 24 hours
SALBUTAMOL (Neb) 2.5 milligrams in 2.5 ml	2.5 milligrams	2.5 milligrams	5 minutes	2.5 ml	No limit
SALBUTAMOL (Neb) 5 milligrams in 2.5 ml	2.5 milligrams	2.5 milligrams	5 minutes	1.25 ml	No limit
TRANEXAMIC ACID (IV) 100 mg/ml	150 mg	NONE	N/A	1.5 ml	150 mg

277

Page for Age

12 MONTHS

Vital Signs

GUIDE WEIGHT	LARYNGEAL MASK	HEART RATE	RESPIRATION RATE	SYSTOLIC BLOOD PRESSURE
10 kg		110–150	25–35	80–95

Airway Size by Type

OROPHARYNGEAL AIRWAY	LARYNGEAL MASK	I-GEL AIRWAY	ENDOTRACHEAL TUBE
00 OR 0	1.5	1.5 OR 2	Diameter: **4.5 mm**; Length: **13 cm**

Defibrillation – Cardiac Arrest

MANUAL	AUTOMATED EXTERNAL DEFIBRILLATOR
40 Joules	A standard AED (either with paediatric attenuation pads or else in paediatric mode) can be used. If paediatric pads are not available, standard adult pads can be used (but must not overlap).

Intravascular Fluid

FLUID	INITIAL DOSE	REPEAT DOSE	DOSE INTERVAL	VOLUME	MAX DOSE
Sodium Chloride (5 ml/kg) (IV/IO) 0.9%	50 ml	50 ml	PRN	50 ml	400 ml
Sodium Chloride (10 ml/kg) (IV/IO) 0.9%	100 ml	100 ml	PRN	100 ml	400 ml
Sodium Chloride (20 ml/kg) (IV/IO) 0.9%	200 ml	200 ml	PRN	200 ml	400 ml

12 MONTHS Page for Age

Cardiac Arrest

DRUG	INITIAL DOSE	REPEAT DOSE	DOSE INTERVAL	VOLUME	MAX DOSE
ADRENALINE **Cardiac Arrest** (IV/IO) 1 milligram in 10 ml (1:10,000)	100 micrograms	100 micrograms	3–5 minutes	1 ml	No limit
AMIODARONE **Cardiac Arrest** (IV/IO) 300 milligrams in 10 ml	50 milligrams (After 3rd shock)	50 milligrams	After 5th shock	1.7 ml	100 milligrams

279

Quick Reference Table — 12 MONTHS — Page for Age

DRUG	INITIAL DOSE	REPEAT DOSE	DOSE INTERVAL	VOLUME	MAX DOSE
ACTIVATED CHARCOAL* (Oral) 50 grams in 250 ml	25 g	25 g	N/A	125 ml	50 grams
ADRENALINE - ANAPHYLAXIS/ASTHMA (IM) 1 milligram in 1 ml (1:1,000)	150 micrograms	150 micrograms	5 minutes	0.15 ml	No limit
BENZYLPENICILLIN (IV/IO) 600 milligrams dissolved in 10 ml water for injection	600 milligrams	NONE	N/A	10 ml	600 milligrams
BENZYLPENICILLIN (IM) 600 milligrams dissolved in 2 ml water for injection	600 milligrams	NONE	N/A	2 ml	600 milligrams
CHLORPHENAMINE (IV/IO/IM) 10 milligrams in 1 ml	2.5 milligrams	NONE	N/A	0.25 ml	2.5 milligrams
CHLORPHENAMINE Oral (tablet)	N/A	N/A	N/A	N/A	N/A
CHLORPHENAMINE Oral (solution) 2 milligrams in 5 ml	1 milligram	NONE	N/A	2.5 ml	1 milligram

*If a large quantity of poison has been ingested, and where there is a risk to life, encourage the child to drink the full dose.

Quick Reference Table

12 MONTHS Page for Age

DRUG	INITIAL DOSE	REPEAT DOSE	DOSE INTERVAL	VOLUME	MAX DOSE
DEXAMETHASONE Oral (solution) 2 milligrams in 5 ml	2 milligrams	NONE	N/A	5 ml	2 milligrams
DEXAMETHASONE Oral (tablet) 2 milligrams per tablet	2 milligrams	NONE	N/A	1 tablet	2 milligrams
DIAZEPAM (IV/IO) 10 milligrams in 2 ml	3 milligrams	3 milligrams	10 minutes	0.6 ml	6 milligrams
DIAZEPAM (Rectal) 5 milligrams in 2.5 ml	5 milligrams	5 milligrams	10 minutes	1 x 5 milligram tube	10 milligrams
GLUCAGON (IM) 1 milligram per vial	500 micrograms	NONE	N/A	0.5 vial	500 micrograms
GLUCOSE 10% (IV) 50 grams in 500 ml	2 grams glucose	2 grams glucose	5 minutes	20 ml	60 ml (6 g glucose)
GLUCOSE 40% ORAL GEL (Buccal) 10 grams in 25 grams of gel	An appropriate amount should be administered, considering the child's size	See initial dose	5 minutes	1 tube	An appropriate amount should be administered, considering the child's size
HYDROCORTISONE (IV/IO/IM) 100 milligrams in 1 ml	50 milligrams	NONE	N/A	0.5 ml	50 milligrams

Quick Reference Table — 12 MONTHS — Page for Age

DRUG	INITIAL DOSE	REPEAT DOSE	DOSE INTERVAL	VOLUME	MAX DOSE
HYDROCORTISONE (IV/IO/IM) 100 milligrams in 2 ml	50 milligrams	NONE	N/A	1 ml	50 milligrams
IBUPROFEN (Oral) 100 milligrams in 5 ml	100 milligrams	100 milligrams	8 hours	5 ml	300 milligrams per 24 hours
IPRATROPIUM BROMIDE (Neb) 250 micrograms in 1 ml	125–250 micrograms	NONE	N/A	0.5–1 ml	125–250 micrograms
IPRATROPIUM BROMIDE (Neb) 500 micrograms in 2 ml	125–250 micrograms	NONE	N/A	0.5–1 ml	125–250 micrograms
MIDAZOLAM** (Buccal) 5 milligrams in 1 ml	5 milligrams	5 milligrams	10 mins	1 ml pre-filled syringe	10 milligrams
MORPHINE SULFATE (IV/IO) 10 milligrams in 10 ml	1 milligram	1 milligram	5 minutes	1 ml	2 milligrams
MORPHINE SULFATE (Oral) 10 milligrams in 5 ml	2 milligrams	NONE	N/A	1 ml	2 milligrams

**Give the dose as prescribed in the child's individual treatment plan/Epilepsy Passport (the dosages described above reflect the recommended dosages for a child of this age).

Quick Reference Table

12 MONTHS Page for Age

DRUG	INITIAL DOSE	REPEAT DOSE	DOSE INTERVAL	VOLUME	MAX DOSE
NALOXONE (IV/IO) 400 micrograms in 1 ml	1,000 micrograms	1,000 micrograms	1 minute	2.5 ml	2,000 micrograms
NALOXONE (IM) 400 micrograms in 1 ml	400 micrograms	400 micrograms	3 minutes	1 ml	2,000 micrograms
ONDANSETRON (IV/IO/IM) 2 milligrams in 1 ml	1 milligram	NONE	N/A	0.5 ml	1 milligram
PARACETAMOL - INFANT SUSPENSION (Oral) 120 milligrams in 5 ml	120 milligrams	120 milligrams	4–6 hours	5 ml	480 milligrams in 24 hours
PARACETAMOL (IV infusion/IO) 10 milligrams in 1 ml	150 milligrams	150 milligrams	4–6 hours	15 ml	600 milligrams in 24 hours
SALBUTAMOL (Neb) 2.5 milligrams in 2.5 ml	2.5 milligrams	2.5 milligrams	5 minutes	2.5 ml	No limit
SALBUTAMOL (Neb) 5 milligrams in 2.5 ml	2.5 milligrams	2.5 milligrams	5 minutes	1.25 ml	No limit
TRANEXAMIC ACID (IV) 100 mg/ml	150 mg	NONE	N/A	1.5 ml	150 mg

18 MONTHS — Page for Age

Vital Signs

GUIDE WEIGHT	HEART RATE	RESPIRATION RATE	SYSTOLIC BLOOD PRESSURE
11 kg	110–150	25–35	80–95

Airway Size by Type

OROPHARYNGEAL AIRWAY	LARYNGEAL MASK	I-GEL AIRWAY	ENDOTRACHEAL TUBE
00 OR 0	2	1.5 OR 2	Diameter: **4.5 mm**; Length: **13 cm**

Defibrillation – Cardiac Arrest

MANUAL	AUTOMATED EXTERNAL DEFIBRILLATOR
50 Joules	A standard AED (either with paediatric attenuation pads or else in paediatric mode) can be used. If paediatric pads are not available, standard adult pads can be used (but must not overlap).

Intravascular Fluid

FLUID	INITIAL DOSE	REPEAT DOSE	DOSE INTERVAL	VOLUME	MAX DOSE
Sodium Chloride (5 ml/kg) (IV/IO) 0.9%	55 ml	55 ml	PRN	55 ml	440 ml
Sodium Chloride (10 ml/kg) (IV/IO) 0.9%	110 ml	110 ml	PRN	110 ml	440 ml
Sodium Chloride (20 ml/kg) (IV/IO) 0.9%	220 ml	220 ml	PRN	220 ml	440 ml

18 MONTHS Page for Age

Cardiac Arrest

DRUG	INITIAL DOSE	REPEAT DOSE	DOSE INTERVAL	VOLUME	MAX DOSE
ADRENALINE **Cardiac Arrest** (IV/IO) 1 milligram in 10 ml (1:10,000)	110 micrograms	110 micrograms	3–5 minutes	1.1 ml	No limit
AMIODARONE **Cardiac Arrest** (IV/IO) 300 milligrams in 10 ml	55 milligrams (After 3rd shock)	55 milligrams	After 5th shock	1.8 ml	110 milligrams

285

Quick Reference Table — 18 MONTHS — Page for Age

DRUG	INITIAL DOSE	REPEAT DOSE	DOSE INTERVAL	VOLUME	MAX DOSE
ACTIVATED CHARCOAL* (Oral) 50 grams in 250 ml	25 g	25 g	N/A	125 ml	50 grams
ADRENALINE - ANAPHYLAXIS/ASTHMA (IM) 1 milligram in 1 ml (1:1,000)	150 micrograms	150 micrograms	5 minutes	0.15 ml	No limit
BENZYLPENICILLIN (IV/IO) 600 milligrams dissolved in 10 ml water for injection	600 milligrams	NONE	N/A	10 ml	600 milligrams
BENZYLPENICILLIN (IM) 600 milligrams dissolved in 2 ml water for injection	600 milligrams	NONE	N/A	2 ml	600 milligrams
CHLORPHENAMINE (IV/IO/IM) 10 milligrams in 1 ml	2.5 milligrams	NONE	N/A	0.25 ml	2.5 milligrams
CHLORPHENAMINE Oral (tablet)	N/A	N/A	N/A	N/A	N/A
CHLORPHENAMINE Oral (solution) 2 milligrams in 5 ml	1 milligram	NONE	N/A	2.5 ml	1 milligram

*If a large quantity of poison has been ingested, and where there is a risk to life, encourage the child to drink the full dose.

Quick Reference Table — 18 MONTHS — Page for Age

DRUG	INITIAL DOSE	REPEAT DOSE	DOSE INTERVAL	VOLUME	MAX DOSE
DEXAMETHASONE Oral (solution) 2 milligrams in 5 ml	2 milligrams	NONE	N/A	5 ml	2 milligrams
DEXAMETHASONE Oral (tablet) 2 milligrams per tablet	2 milligrams	NONE	N/A	1 tablet	2 milligrams
DIAZEPAM IV/IO 10 milligrams in 2 ml	3.5 milligrams	3.5 milligrams	10 minutes	0.7 ml	7 milligrams
DIAZEPAM Rectal 5 milligrams in 2.5 ml	5 milligrams	5 milligrams	10 minutes	1 x 5 milligram tube	10 milligrams
GLUCAGON IM 1 milligram per vial	500 micrograms	NONE	N/A	0.5 vial	500 micrograms
GLUCOSE 10% IV 50 grams in 500 ml	2 grams glucose	2 grams glucose	5 minutes	20 ml	60 ml (6 g glucose)
GLUCOSE 40% ORAL GEL Buccal 10 grams in 25 grams of gel	An appropriate amount should be administered, considering the child's size	See initial dose	5 minutes	1 tube	An appropriate amount should be administered, considering the child's size
HYDROCORTISONE IV/IO/IM 100 milligrams in 1 ml	50 milligrams	NONE	N/A	0.5 ml	50 milligrams

Quick Reference Table — **18 MONTHS** — Page for Age

DRUG	INITIAL DOSE	REPEAT DOSE	DOSE INTERVAL	VOLUME	MAX DOSE
HYDROCORTISONE (IV/IO/IM) 100 milligrams in 2 ml	50 milligrams	NONE	N/A	1 ml	50 milligrams
IBUPROFEN (Oral) 100 milligrams in 5 ml	100 milligrams	100 milligrams	8 hours	5 ml	300 milligrams per 24 hours
IPRATROPIUM BROMIDE (Neb) 250 micrograms in 1 ml	250 micrograms	NONE	N/A	1 ml	250 micrograms
IPRATROPIUM BROMIDE (Neb) 500 micrograms in 2 ml	250 micrograms	NONE	N/A	1 ml	250 micrograms
MIDAZOLAM** (Buccal) 5 milligrams in 1 ml	5 milligrams	5 milligrams	10 mins	1 ml pre-filled syringe	10 milligrams
MORPHINE SULFATE (IV/IO) 10 milligrams in 10 ml	1 milligram	1 milligram	5 minutes	1 ml	2 milligrams
MORPHINE SULFATE (Oral) 10 milligrams in 5 ml	2 milligrams	NONE	N/A	1 ml	2 milligrams
NALOXONE (IV/IO) 400 micrograms in 1 ml	1,000 micrograms	1,000 micrograms	1 minute	2.5 ml	2,000 micrograms

**Give the dose as prescribed in the child's individual treatment plan/Epilepsy Passport (the dosages described above reflect the recommended dosages for a child of this age).

Quick Reference Table

18 MONTHS — Page for Age

DRUG	INITIAL DOSE	REPEAT DOSE	DOSE INTERVAL	VOLUME	MAX DOSE
NALOXONE (IM) 400 micrograms in 1 ml	400 micrograms	400 micrograms	3 minutes	1 ml	2,000 micrograms
ONDANSETRON (IV/IO/IM) 2 milligrams in 1 ml	1 milligram	NONE	N/A	0.5 ml	1 milligram
PARACETAMOL - INFANT SUSPENSION (Oral) 120 milligrams in 5 ml	120 milligrams	120 milligrams	4–6 hours	5 ml	480 milligrams in 24 hours
PARACETAMOL (IV infusion/IO) 10 milligrams in 1 ml	150 milligrams	150 milligrams	4–6 hours	15 ml	600 milligrams in 24 hours
SALBUTAMOL (Neb) 2.5 milligrams in 2.5 ml	2.5 milligrams	2.5 milligrams	5 minutes	2.5 ml	No limit
SALBUTAMOL (Neb) 5 milligrams in 2.5 ml	2.5 milligrams	2.5 milligrams	5 minutes	1.25 ml	No limit
TRANEXAMIC ACID (IV) 100 mg/ml	150 mg	NONE	N/A	1.5 ml	150 mg

289

Page for Age

2 YEARS

Vital Signs

GUIDE WEIGHT	LARYNGEAL MASK	HEART RATE	RESPIRATION RATE	SYSTOLIC BLOOD PRESSURE
12 kg		95–140	25–30	80–100

Airway Size by Type

OROPHARYNGEAL AIRWAY	LARYNGEAL MASK	I-GEL AIRWAY	ENDOTRACHEAL TUBE
0 OR 1	2	1.5 OR 2	Diameter: **5 mm**; Length: **14 cm**

Defibrillation – Cardiac Arrest

MANUAL	AUTOMATED EXTERNAL DEFIBRILLATOR
50 Joules	A standard AED (either with paediatric attenuation pads or else in paediatric mode) can be used. If paediatric pads are not available, standard adult pads can be used (but must not overlap).

Intravascular Fluid

FLUID	INITIAL DOSE	REPEAT DOSE	DOSE INTERVAL	VOLUME	MAX DOSE
Sodium Chloride (5 ml/kg) (IV/IO) 0.9%	60 ml	60 ml	PRN	60 ml	480 ml
Sodium Chloride (10 ml/kg) (IV/IO) 0.9%	120 ml	120 ml	PRN	120 ml	480 ml
Sodium Chloride (20 ml/kg) (IV/IO) 0.9%	240 ml	240 ml	PRN	240 ml	480 ml

Cardiac Arrest

2 YEARS — Page for Age

DRUG	INITIAL DOSE	REPEAT DOSE	DOSE INTERVAL	VOLUME	MAX DOSE
ADRENALINE **Cardiac Arrest** (IV/IO) 1 milligram in 10 ml (1:10,000)	120 micrograms	120 micrograms	3–5 minutes	1.2 ml	No limit
AMIODARONE **Cardiac Arrest** (IV/IO) 300 milligrams in 10 ml	60 milligrams (After 3rd shock)	60 milligrams	After 5th shock	2 ml	120 milligrams

Quick Reference Table — 2 YEARS — Page for Age

DRUG	INITIAL DOSE	REPEAT DOSE	DOSE INTERVAL	VOLUME	MAX DOSE
ACTIVATED CHARCOAL* (Oral) 50 grams in 250 ml	25 g	25 g	N/A	125 ml	50 grams
ADRENALINE - ANAPHYLAXIS/ ASTHMA (IM) 1 milligram in 1 ml (1:1,000)	150 micrograms	150 micrograms	5 minutes	0.15 ml	No limit
BENZYLPENICILLIN (IV/IO) 600 milligrams dissolved in 10 ml water for injection	600 milligrams	NONE	N/A	10 ml	600 milligrams
BENZYLPENICILLIN (IM) 600 milligrams dissolved in 2 ml water for injection	600 milligrams	NONE	N/A	2 ml	600 milligrams
CHLORPHENAMINE (IV/IO/IM) 10 milligrams in 1 ml	2.5 milligrams	NONE	N/A	0.25 ml	2.5 milligrams
CHLORPHENAMINE Oral (tablet)	N/A	N/A	N/A	N/A	N/A

*If a large quantity of poison has been ingested, and where there is a risk to life, encourage the child to drink the full dose.

Quick Reference Table

2 YEARS

Page for Age

DRUG	INITIAL DOSE	REPEAT DOSE	DOSE INTERVAL	VOLUME	MAX DOSE
CHLORPHENAMINE Oral (solution) 2 milligrams in 5 ml	1 milligram	NONE	N/A	2.5 ml	1 milligram
DEXAMETHASONE Oral (solution) 2 milligrams in 5 ml	2 milligrams	NONE	N/A	5 ml	2 milligrams
DEXAMETHASONE Oral (tablet) 2 milligrams per tablet	2 milligrams	NONE	N/A	1 tablet	2 milligrams
DIAZEPAM (IV/IO) 10 milligrams in 2 ml	4 milligrams	4 milligrams	10 minutes	0.8 ml	8 milligrams
DIAZEPAM (Rectal) 5 milligrams in 2.5 ml	5 milligrams	5 milligrams	10 minutes	1 x 5 milligram tube	10 milligrams
GLUCAGON (IM) 1 milligram per vial	500 micrograms	NONE	N/A	0.5 vial	500 micrograms
GLUCOSE 10% (IV) 50 grams in 500 ml	2.5 grams glucose	2.5 grams glucose	5 minutes	25 ml	75 ml (7.5 g glucose)

293

Quick Reference Table — 2 YEARS — Page for Age

DRUG	INITIAL DOSE	REPEAT DOSE	DOSE INTERVAL	VOLUME	MAX DOSE
GLUCOSE 40% ORAL GEL (Buccal) 10 grams in 25 grams of gel	10 grams	10 grams	5 minutes	1 tube	2 tubes/20 grams
HYDROCORTISONE (IV/IO/IM) 100 milligrams in 1 ml	50 milligrams	NONE	N/A	0.5 ml	50 milligrams
HYDROCORTISONE (IV/IO/IM) 100 milligrams in 2 ml	50 milligrams	NONE	N/A	1 ml	50 milligrams
IBUPROFEN (Oral) 100 milligrams in 5 ml	100 milligrams	100 milligrams	8 hours	5 ml	300 milligrams per 24 hours
IPRATROPIUM BROMIDE (Neb) 250 micrograms in 1 ml	250 micrograms	NONE	N/A	1 ml	250 micrograms
IPRATROPIUM BROMIDE (Neb) 500 micrograms in 2 ml	250 micrograms	NONE	N/A	1 ml	250 micrograms

Quick Reference Table

2 YEARS

Page for Age

DRUG	INITIAL DOSE	REPEAT DOSE	DOSE INTERVAL	VOLUME	MAX DOSE
MIDAZOLAM** (Buccal) 5 milligrams in 1 ml	5 milligrams	5 milligrams	10 mins	1 ml pre-filled syringe	10 milligrams
MORPHINE SULFATE (IV/IO) 10 milligrams in 10 ml	1 milligram	1 milligram	5 minutes	1 ml	2 milligrams
MORPHINE SULFATE (Oral) 10 milligrams in 5 ml	2 milligrams	NONE	N/A	1 ml	2 milligrams
NALOXONE (IV/IO) 400 micrograms in 1 ml	800 micrograms	800 micrograms	1 minute	3 ml	2,000 micrograms
NALOXONE (IM) 400 micrograms in 1 ml	1,200 micrograms	400 micrograms	3 minutes	1 ml	2,000 micrograms
ONDANSETRON (IV/IO/IM) 2 milligrams in 1 ml	1 milligram	NONE	N/A	0.5 ml	1 milligram

Give the dose as prescribed in the child's individual treatment plan/Epilepsy Passport (the dosages described above reflect the recommended dosages for a child of this age).

295

Quick Reference Table

2 YEARS

Page for Age

DRUG	INITIAL DOSE	REPEAT DOSE	DOSE INTERVAL	VOLUME	MAX DOSE
PARACETAMOL - INFANT SUSPENSION (Oral) 120 milligrams in 5 ml	180 milligrams	180 milligrams	4–6 hours	7.5 ml	720 milligrams in 24 hours
PARACETAMOL (IV infusion/IO) 10 milligrams in 1 ml	200 milligrams	200 milligrams	4–6 hours	20 ml	800 milligrams in 24 hours
SALBUTAMOL (Neb) 2.5 milligrams in 2.5 ml	2.5 milligrams	2.5 milligrams	5 minutes	2.5 ml	No limit
SALBUTAMOL (Neb) 5 milligrams in 2.5 ml	2.5 milligrams	2.5 milligrams	5 minutes	1.25 ml	No limit
TRANEXAMIC ACID (IV) 100 mg/ml	200 mg	NONE	N/A	2 ml	200 mg

This page left intentionally blank for your notes

Page for Age

3 YEARS

Vital Signs

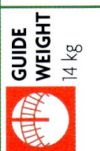

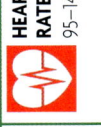

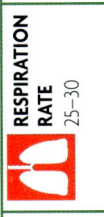

GUIDE WEIGHT	HEART RATE	RESPIRATION RATE	SYSTOLIC BLOOD PRESSURE
14 kg	95–140	25–30	80–100

Airway Size by Type

OROPHARYNGEAL AIRWAY	LARYNGEAL MASK	I-GEL AIRWAY	ENDOTRACHEAL TUBE
1	2	2	Diameter: **5 mm**; Length: **14 cm**

Defibrillation – Cardiac Arrest

MANUAL	AUTOMATED EXTERNAL DEFIBRILLATOR
60 Joules	A standard AED (either with paediatric attenuation pads or else in paediatric mode) can be used. If paediatric pads are not available, standard adult pads can be used (but must not overlap).

Intravascular Fluid

FLUID	INITIAL DOSE	REPEAT DOSE	DOSE INTERVAL	VOLUME	MAX DOSE
Sodium Chloride (5 ml/kg) 0.9% (IV/IO)	70 ml	70 ml	PRN	70 ml	560 ml
Sodium Chloride (10 ml/kg) 0.9% (IV/IO)	140 ml	140 ml	PRN	140 ml	560 ml
Sodium Chloride (20 ml/kg) 0.9% (IV/IO)	280 ml	280 ml	PRN	280 ml	560 ml

Cardiac Arrest

3 YEARS — Page for Age

DRUG	INITIAL DOSE	REPEAT DOSE	DOSE INTERVAL	VOLUME	MAX DOSE
ADRENALINE **Cardiac Arrest** (IV/IO) 1 milligram in 10 ml (1:10,000)	140 micrograms	140 micrograms	3–5 minutes	1.4 ml	No limit
AMIODARONE **Cardiac Arrest** (IV/IO) 300 milligrams in 10 ml	70 milligrams (After 3rd shock)	70 milligrams	After 5th shock	2.3 ml	140 milligrams

Quick Reference Table — 3 YEARS — Page for Age

DRUG	INITIAL DOSE	REPEAT DOSE	DOSE INTERVAL	VOLUME	MAX DOSE
ACTIVATED CHARCOAL* (Oral) 50 grams in 250 ml	25 g	25 g	N/A	125 ml	50 grams
ADRENALINE - ANAPHYLAXIS/ASTHMA (IM) 1 milligram in 1 ml (1:1,000)	150 micrograms	150 micrograms	5 minutes	0.15 ml	No limit
BENZYLPENICILLIN (IV/IO) 600 milligrams dissolved in 10 ml water for injection	600 milligrams	NONE	N/A	10 ml	600 milligrams
BENZYLPENICILLIN (IM) 600 milligrams dissolved in 2 ml water for injection	600 milligrams	NONE	N/A	2 ml	600 milligrams
CHLORPHENAMINE (IV/IO/IM) 10 milligrams in 1 ml	2.5 milligrams	NONE	N/A	0.25 ml	2.5 milligrams
CHLORPHENAMINE Oral (tablet)	N/A	N/A	N/A	N/A	N/A
CHLORPHENAMINE Oral (solution) 2 milligrams in 5 ml	1 milligram	NONE	N/A	2.5 ml	1 milligram

*If a large quantity of poison has been ingested, and where there is a risk to life, encourage the child to drink the full dose.

Quick Reference Table

3 YEARS — Page for Age

DRUG	INITIAL DOSE	REPEAT DOSE	DOSE INTERVAL	VOLUME	MAX DOSE
DEXAMETHASONE Oral (solution) 2 milligrams in 5 ml	2.4 milligrams	NONE	N/A	6 ml	2.4 milligrams
DEXAMETHASONE Oral (tablet) 2 milligrams per tablet	2 milligrams	NONE	N/A	1 tablet	2 milligrams
DIAZEPAM (IV/IO) 10 milligrams in 2 ml	4.5 milligrams	4.5 milligrams	10 minutes	0.9 ml	9 milligrams
DIAZEPAM (Rectal) 5 milligrams in 2.5 ml	5 milligrams	5 milligrams	10 minutes	1 x 5 milligram tube	10 milligrams
GLUCAGON (IM) 1 milligram per vial	500 micrograms	NONE	N/A	0.5 vial	500 micrograms
GLUCOSE 10% (IV) 50 grams in 500 ml	3 grams glucose	3 grams glucose	5 minutes	30 ml	90 ml (9 g glucose)
GLUCOSE 40% ORAL GEL (Buccal) 10 grams in 25 grams of gel	10 grams	10 grams	5 minutes	1 tube	2 tubes/20 grams
HYDROCORTISONE (IV/IO/IM) 100 milligrams in 1 ml	50 milligrams	NONE	N/A	0.5 ml	50 milligrams

Quick Reference Table — 3 YEARS — Page for Age

DRUG	INITIAL DOSE	REPEAT DOSE	DOSE INTERVAL	VOLUME	MAX DOSE
HYDROCORTISONE (IV/IO/IM) 100 milligrams in 2 ml	50 milligrams	NONE	N/A	1 ml	50 milligrams
IBUPROFEN (Oral) 100 milligrams in 5 ml	100 milligrams	100 milligrams	8 hours	5 ml	300 milligrams per 24 hours
IPRATROPIUM BROMIDE (Neb) 250 micrograms in 1 ml	250 micrograms	NONE	N/A	1 ml	250 micrograms
IPRATROPIUM BROMIDE (Neb) 500 micrograms in 2 ml	250 micrograms	NONE	N/A	1 ml	250 micrograms
MIDAZOLAM** (Buccal) 5 milligrams in 1 ml	5 milligrams	5 milligrams	10 mins	1 ml pre-filled syringe	10 milligrams
MORPHINE SULFATE (IV/IO) 10 milligrams in 10 ml	1.5 milligrams	1.5 milligrams	5 minutes	1.5 ml	3 milligrams
MORPHINE SULFATE (Oral) 10 milligrams in 5 ml	3 milligrams	NONE	N/A	1.5 ml	3 milligrams
NALOXONE (IV/IO) 400 micrograms in 1 ml	1,200 micrograms	800 micrograms	1 minute	3 ml	2,000 micrograms

**Give the dose as prescribed in the child's individual treatment plan/Epilepsy Passport (the dosages described above reflect the recommended dosages for a child of this age).

Quick Reference Table

3 YEARS Page for Age

DRUG	INITIAL DOSE	REPEAT DOSE	DOSE INTERVAL	VOLUME	MAX DOSE
NALOXONE (IM) 400 micrograms in 1 ml	400 micrograms	400 micrograms	3 minutes	1 ml	2,000 micrograms
ONDANSETRON (IV/IO/IM) 2 milligrams in 1 ml	1.5 milligrams	NONE	N/A	0.75 ml	1.5 milligrams
PARACETAMOL - INFANT SUSPENSION (Oral) 120 milligrams in 5 ml	180 milligrams	180 milligrams	4–6 hours	7.5 ml	720 milligrams in 24 hours
PARACETAMOL (IV infusion/IO) 10 milligrams in 1 ml	200 milligrams	200 milligrams	4–6 hours	20 ml	800 milligrams in 24 hours
SALBUTAMOL (Neb) 2.5 milligrams in 2.5 ml	2.5 milligrams	2.5 milligrams	5 minutes	2.5 ml	No limit
SALBUTAMOL (Neb) 5 milligrams in 2.5 ml	2.5 milligrams	2.5 milligrams	5 minutes	1.25 ml	No limit
TRANEXAMIC ACID (IV) 100 mg/ml	200 mg	NONE	N/A	2 ml	200 mg

303

Page for Age

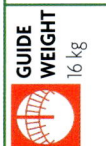

4 YEARS

Vital Signs

GUIDE WEIGHT	HEART RATE	RESPIRATION RATE	SYSTOLIC BLOOD PRESSURE
16 kg	95–140	25–30	80–100

Airway Size by Type

OROPHARYNGEAL AIRWAY	LARYNGEAL MASK	I-GEL AIRWAY	ENDOTRACHEAL TUBE
1	2	2	Diameter: **5 mm**; Length: **15 cm**

Defibrillation – Cardiac Arrest

MANUAL	AUTOMATED EXTERNAL DEFIBRILLATOR
70 Joules	A standard AED (either with paediatric attenuation pads or else in paediatric mode) can be used. If paediatric pads are not available, standard adult pads can be used (but must not overlap).

Intravascular Fluid

FLUID	INITIAL DOSE	REPEAT DOSE	DOSE INTERVAL	VOLUME	MAX DOSE
Sodium Chloride (5 ml/kg) (IV/IO) 0.9%	80 ml	80 ml	PRN	80 ml	640 ml
Sodium Chloride (10 ml/kg) (IV/IO) 0.9%	160 ml	160 ml	PRN	160 ml	640 ml
Sodium Chloride (20 ml/kg) (IV/IO) 0.9%	320 ml	320 ml	PRN	320 ml	640 ml

Cardiac Arrest

4 YEARS — Page for Age

DRUG	INITIAL DOSE	REPEAT DOSE	DOSE INTERVAL	VOLUME	MAX DOSE
ADRENALINE Cardiac Arrest (IV/IO) 1 milligram in 10 ml (1:10,000)	160 micrograms	160 micrograms	3–5 minutes	1.6 ml	No limit
AMIODARONE Cardiac Arrest (IV/IO) 300 milligrams in 10 ml	80 milligrams (After 3rd shock)	80 milligrams	After 5th shock	2.7 ml	160 milligrams

305

Quick Reference Table — 4 YEARS — Page for Age

DRUG	INITIAL DOSE	REPEAT DOSE	DOSE INTERVAL	VOLUME	MAX DOSE
ACTIVATED CHARCOAL* (Oral) 50 grams in 250 ml	25 g	25 g	N/A	125 ml	50 grams
ADRENALINE - ANAPHYLAXIS/ASTHMA (IM) 1 milligram in 1 ml (1:1,000)	150 micrograms	150 micrograms	5 minutes	0.15 ml	No limit
BENZYLPENICILLIN (IV/IO) 600 milligrams dissolved in 10 ml water for injection	600 milligrams	NONE	N/A	10 ml	600 milligrams
BENZYLPENICILLIN (IM) 600 milligrams dissolved in 2 ml water for injection	600 milligrams	NONE	N/A	2 ml	600 milligrams
CHLORPHENAMINE (IV/IO/IM) 10 milligrams in 1 ml	2.5 milligrams	NONE	N/A	0.25 ml	2.5 milligrams
CHLORPHENAMINE Oral (tablet)	N/A	N/A	N/A	N/A	N/A
CHLORPHENAMINE Oral (solution) 2 milligrams in 5 ml	1 milligram	NONE	N/A	2.5 ml	1 milligram

*If a large quantity of poison has been ingested, and where there is a risk to life, encourage the child to drink the full dose.

Quick Reference Table

4 YEARS Page for Age

DRUG	INITIAL DOSE	REPEAT DOSE	DOSE INTERVAL	VOLUME	MAX DOSE
DEXAMETHASONE Oral (solution) 2 milligrams in 5 ml	3.2 milligrams	NONE	N/A	8 ml	3.2 milligrams
DEXAMETHASONE Oral (tablet) 2 milligrams per tablet	4 milligrams	NONE	N/A	2 tablets	4 milligrams
DIAZEPAM (IV/IO) 10 milligrams in 2 ml	5 milligrams	5 milligrams	10 minutes	1 ml	10 milligrams
DIAZEPAM (Rectal) 5 milligrams in 2.5 ml	5 milligrams	5 milligrams	10 minutes	1 x 5 milligram tube	10 milligrams
GLUCAGON (IM) 1 milligram per vial	500 micrograms	NONE	N/A	0.5 vial	500 micrograms
GLUCOSE 10% (IV) 50 grams in 500 ml	3 grams glucose	3 grams glucose	5 minutes	30 ml	90 ml (9 g glucose)
GLUCOSE 40% ORAL GEL (Buccal) 10 grams in 25 grams of gel	10 grams	10 grams	5 minutes	1 tube	2 tubes/20 grams
HYDROCORTISONE (IV/IO/IM) 100 milligrams in 1 ml	50 milligrams	NONE	N/A	0.5 ml	50 milligrams

307

Quick Reference Table — 4 YEARS — Page for Age

DRUG	INITIAL DOSE	REPEAT DOSE	DOSE INTERVAL	VOLUME	MAX DOSE
HYDROCORTISONE (IV/IO/IM) 100 milligrams in 2 ml	50 milligrams	NONE	N/A	1 ml	50 milligrams
IBUPROFEN (Oral) 100 milligrams in 5 ml	150 milligrams	150 milligrams	8 hours	7.5 ml	450 milligrams per 24 hours
IPRATROPIUM BROMIDE (Neb) 250 micrograms in 1 ml	250 micrograms	NONE	N/A	1 ml	250 micrograms
IPRATROPIUM BROMIDE (Neb) 500 micrograms in 2 ml	250 micrograms	NONE	N/A	1 ml	250 micrograms
MIDAZOLAM** (Buccal) 5 milligrams in 1 ml	5 milligrams	5 milligrams	10 mins	1 ml pre-filled syringe	10 milligrams
MORPHINE SULFATE (IV/IO) 10 milligrams in 10 ml	1.5 milligrams	1.5 milligrams	5 minutes	1.5 ml	3 milligrams
MORPHINE SULFATE (Oral) 10 milligrams in 5 ml	3 milligrams	NONE	N/A	1.5 ml	3 milligrams
NALOXONE (IV/IO) 400 micrograms in 1 ml	1,600 micrograms	400 micrograms	1 minute	4 ml	2,000 micrograms

**Give the dose as prescribed in the child's individual treatment plan/Epilepsy Passport (the dosages described above reflect the recommended dosages for a child of this age).

Quick Reference Table

4 YEARS Page for Age

DRUG	INITIAL DOSE	REPEAT DOSE	DOSE INTERVAL	VOLUME	MAX DOSE
NALOXONE (IM) 400 micrograms in 1 ml	400 micrograms	400 micrograms	3 minutes	1 ml	2,000 micrograms
ONDANSETRON (IV/IO/IM) 2 milligrams in 1 ml	1.5 milligrams	NONE	N/A	0.75 ml	1.5 milligrams
PARACETAMOL - INFANT SUSPENSION (Oral) 120 milligrams in 5 ml	240 milligrams	240 milligrams	4–6 hours	10 ml	960 milligrams in 24 hours
PARACETAMOL (IV infusion/IO) 10 milligrams in 1 ml	250 milligrams	250 milligrams	4–6 hours	25 ml	1 gram in 24 hours
SALBUTAMOL (Neb) 2.5 milligrams in 2.5 ml	2.5 milligrams	2.5 milligrams	5 minutes	2.5 ml	No limit
SALBUTAMOL (Neb) 5 milligrams in 2.5 ml	2.5 milligrams	2.5 milligrams	5 minutes	1.25 ml	No limit
TRANEXAMIC ACID (IV) 100 mg/ml	250 mg	NONE	N/A	2.5 ml	250 mg

309

Page for Age

5 YEARS

Vital Signs

GUIDE WEIGHT	HEART RATE	RESPIRATION RATE	SYSTOLIC BLOOD PRESSURE
19 kg	80–120	20–25	90–100

Airway Size by Type

OROPHARYNGEAL AIRWAY	LARYNGEAL MASK	I-GEL AIRWAY	ENDOTRACHEAL TUBE
1	2	2	Diameter: **5.5 mm**; Length: **15 cm**

Defibrillation – Cardiac Arrest

MANUAL	AUTOMATED EXTERNAL DEFIBRILLATOR
80 Joules	A standard AED (either with paediatric attenuation pads or else in paediatric mode) can be used. If paediatric pads are not available, standard adult pads can be used (but must not overlap).

Intravascular Fluid

FLUID	INITIAL DOSE	REPEAT DOSE	DOSE INTERVAL	VOLUME	MAX DOSE
Sodium Chloride (5 ml/kg) 0.9% (IV/IO)	95 ml	95 ml	PRN	95 ml	760 ml
Sodium Chloride (10 ml/kg) 0.9% (IV/IO)	190 ml	190 ml	PRN	190 ml	760 ml
Sodium Chloride (20 ml/kg) 0.9% (IV/IO)	380 ml	380 ml	PRN	380 ml	760 ml

Cardiac Arrest

5 YEARS
Page for Age

DRUG	INITIAL DOSE	REPEAT DOSE	DOSE INTERVAL	VOLUME	MAX DOSE
ADRENALINE **Cardiac Arrest** (IV/IO) 1 milligram in 10 ml (1:10,000)	190 micrograms	190 micrograms	3–5 minutes	1.9 ml	No limit
AMIODARONE **Cardiac Arrest** (IV/IO) 300 milligrams in 10 ml	100 milligrams (After 3rd shock)	100 milligrams	After 5th shock	3.3 ml	200 milligrams

311

Quick Reference Table — 5 YEARS — Page for Age

DRUG	INITIAL DOSE	REPEAT DOSE	DOSE INTERVAL	VOLUME	MAX DOSE
ACTIVATED CHARCOAL* (Oral) 50 grams in 250 ml	25 g	25 g	N/A	125 ml	50 grams
ADRENALINE - ANAPHYLAXIS/ASTHMA (IM) 1 milligram in 1 ml (1:1,000)	150 micrograms	150 micrograms	5 minutes	0.15 ml	No limit
BENZYLPENICILLIN (IV/IO) 600 milligrams dissolved in 10 ml water for injection	600 milligrams	NONE	N/A	10 ml	600 milligrams
BENZYLPENICILLIN (IM) 600 milligrams dissolved in 2 ml water for injection	600 milligrams	NONE	N/A	2 ml	600 milligrams
CHLORPHENAMINE (IV/IO/IM) 10 milligrams in 1 ml	2.5 milligrams	NONE	N/A	0.25 ml	2.5 milligrams
CHLORPHENAMINE Oral (tablet)	N/A	N/A	N/A	N/A	N/A
CHLORPHENAMINE Oral (solution) 2 milligrams in 5 ml	1 milligram	NONE	N/A	2.5 ml	1 milligram

*If a large quantity of poison has been ingested, and where there is a risk to life, encourage the child to drink the full dose.

Quick Reference Table

5 YEARS — Page for Age

DRUG	INITIAL DOSE	REPEAT DOSE	DOSE INTERVAL	VOLUME	MAX DOSE
DEXAMETHASONE Oral (solution) 2 milligrams in 5 ml	3.2 milligrams	NONE	N/A	8 ml	3.2 milligrams
DEXAMETHASONE Oral (tablet) 2 milligrams per tablet	4 milligrams	NONE	N/A	2 tablets	4 milligrams
DIAZEPAM (IV/IO) 10 milligrams in 2 ml	6 milligrams	6 milligrams	10 minutes	1.2 ml	12 milligrams
DIAZEPAM (Rectal) 10 milligrams in 2.5 ml	10 milligrams	10 milligrams	10 minutes	1 x 10 milligram tube	20 milligrams
GLUCAGON (IM) 1 milligram per vial	500 micrograms	NONE	N/A	0.5 vial	500 micrograms
GLUCOSE 10% (IV) 50 grams in 500 ml	4 grams glucose	4 grams glucose	5 minutes	40 ml	120 ml (12 g glucose)
GLUCOSE 40% ORAL GEL (Buccal) 10 grams in 25 grams of gel	10 grams	10 grams	5 minutes	1 tube	2 tubes/20 grams
HYDROCORTISONE (IV/IO/IM) 100 milligrams in 1 ml	50 milligrams	NONE	N/A	0.5 ml	50 milligrams

Quick Reference Table — 5 YEARS — Page for Age

DRUG	INITIAL DOSE	REPEAT DOSE	DOSE INTERVAL	VOLUME	MAX DOSE
HYDROCORTISONE (IV/IO/IM) 100 milligrams in 2 ml	50 milligrams	NONE	N/A	1 ml	50 milligrams
IBUPROFEN (Oral) 100 milligrams in 5 ml	150 milligrams	150 milligrams	8 hours	7.5 ml	450 milligrams per 24 hours
IPRATROPIUM BROMIDE (Neb) 250 micrograms in 1 ml	250 micrograms	NONE	N/A	1 ml	250 micrograms
IPRATROPIUM BROMIDE (Neb) 500 micrograms in 2 ml	250 micrograms	NONE	N/A	1 ml	250 micrograms
MIDAZOLAM** (Buccal) 5 milligrams in 1 ml	7.5 milligrams	7.5 milligrams	10 mins	1.5 ml pre-filled syringe	15 milligrams
MORPHINE SULFATE (IV/IO) 10 milligrams in 10 ml	2 milligrams	2 milligrams	5 minutes	2 ml	4 milligrams
MORPHINE SULFATE (Oral) 10 milligrams in 5 ml	4 milligrams	NONE	N/A	2 ml	4 milligrams
NALOXONE (IV/IO) 400 micrograms in 1 ml	2,000 micrograms	Seek advice	N/A	5 ml	2,000 micrograms

**Give the dose as prescribed in the child's individual treatment plan/Epilepsy Passport (the dosages described above reflect the recommended dosages for a child of this age).

PAGE AGE

Quick Reference Table

5 YEARS — Page for Age

DRUG	INITIAL DOSE	REPEAT DOSE	DOSE INTERVAL	VOLUME	MAX DOSE
NALOXONE (IM) 400 micrograms in 1 ml	400 micrograms	400 micrograms	3 minutes	1 ml	2,000 micrograms
ONDANSETRON (IV/IO/IM) 2 milligrams in 1 ml	2 milligrams	NONE	N/A	1 ml	2 milligrams
PARACETAMOL - INFANT SUSPENSION (Oral) 120 milligrams in 5 ml	240 milligrams	240 milligrams	4–6 hours	10 ml	960 milligrams in 24 hours
PARACETAMOL (IV infusion/IO) 10 milligrams in 1 ml	300 milligrams	300 milligrams	4–6 hours	30 ml	1.2 gram in 24 hours
SALBUTAMOL (Neb) 2.5 milligrams in 2.5 ml	2.5 milligrams	2.5 milligrams	5 minutes	2.5 ml	No limit
SALBUTAMOL (Neb) 5 milligrams in 2.5 ml	2.5 milligrams	2.5 milligrams	5 minutes	1.25 ml	No limit
TRANEXAMIC ACID (IV) 100 mg/ml	300 mg	NONE	N/A	3 ml	300 mg

RESUS PAED GENERAL MEDICAL TRAUMA SP SITU MATERNITY MEDS PAGE AGE

Page for Age

6 YEARS

Vital Signs

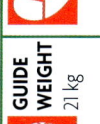

GUIDE WEIGHT	LARYNGEAL MASK	HEART RATE	RESPIRATION RATE	SYSTOLIC BLOOD PRESSURE
21 kg		80–120	20–25	90–110

Airway Size by Type

OROPHARYNGEAL AIRWAY	LARYNGEAL MASK	I-GEL AIRWAY	ENDOTRACHEAL TUBE
1	2.5	2	Diameter: **6 mm**; Length: **16 cm**

Defibrillation – Cardiac Arrest

MANUAL	AUTOMATED EXTERNAL DEFIBRILLATOR
80 Joules	A standard AED (either with paediatric attenuation pads or else in paediatric mode) can be used. If paediatric pads are not available, standard adult pads can be used (but must not overlap).

Intravascular Fluid

FLUID	INITIAL DOSE	REPEAT DOSE	DOSE INTERVAL	VOLUME	MAX DOSE
Sodium Chloride (5 ml/kg) 0.9% (IV/IO)	105 ml	105 ml	PRN	105 ml	840 ml
Sodium Chloride (10 ml/kg) 0.9% (IV/IO)	210 ml	210 ml	PRN	210 ml	840 ml
Sodium Chloride (20 ml/kg) 0.9% (IV/IO)	420 ml	420 ml	PRN	420 ml	840 ml

Cardiac Arrest

6 YEARS Page for Age

DRUG	INITIAL DOSE	REPEAT DOSE	DOSE INTERVAL	VOLUME	MAX DOSE
ADRENALINE **Cardiac Arrest** (IV/IO) 1 milligram in 10 ml (1:10,000)	210 micrograms	210 micrograms	3–5 minutes	2.1 ml	No limit
AMIODARONE **Cardiac Arrest** (IV/IO) 300 milligrams in 10 ml	100 milligrams (After 3rd shock)	100 milligrams	After 5th shock	3.3 ml	200 milligrams

Quick Reference Table — 6 YEARS — Page for Age

DRUG	INITIAL DOSE	REPEAT DOSE	DOSE INTERVAL	VOLUME	MAX DOSE
ACTIVATED CHARCOAL* (Oral) 50 grams in 250 ml	25 g	25 g	N/A	125 ml	50 grams
ADRENALINE - ANAPHYLAXIS/ASTHMA (IM) 1 milligram in 1 ml (1:1,000)	300 micrograms	300 micrograms	5 minutes	0.3 ml	No limit
BENZYLPENICILLIN (IV/IO) 600 milligrams dissolved in 10 ml water for injection	600 milligrams	NONE	N/A	10 ml	600 milligrams
BENZYLPENICILLIN (IM) 600 milligrams dissolved in 2 ml water for injection	600 milligrams	NONE	N/A	2 ml	600 milligrams
CHLORPHENAMINE (IV/IO/IM) 10 milligrams in 1 ml	5 milligrams	NONE	N/A	0.5 ml	5 milligrams
CHLORPHENAMINE Oral (tablet) 4 milligrams per tablet	2 milligrams	NONE	N/A	½ of one tablet	2 milligrams
CHLORPHENAMINE Oral (solution) 2 milligrams in 5 ml	2 milligrams	NONE	N/A	5 ml	2 milligrams

*If a large quantity of poison has been ingested, and where there is a risk to life, encourage the child to drink the full dose.

Quick Reference Table — 6 YEARS Page for Age

DRUG	INITIAL DOSE	REPEAT DOSE	DOSE INTERVAL	VOLUME	MAX DOSE
DEXAMETHASONE Oral (solution) 2 milligrams in 5 ml	3.2 milligrams	NONE	N/A	8 ml	3.2 milligrams
DEXAMETHASONE Oral (tablet) 2 milligrams per tablet	4 milligrams	NONE	N/A	2 tablets	4 milligrams
DIAZEPAM (IV/IO) 10 milligrams in 2 ml	6.5 milligrams	6.5 milligrams	10 minutes	1.3 ml	13 milligrams
DIAZEPAM (Rectal) 10 milligrams in 2.5 ml	10 milligrams	10 milligrams	10 minutes	1 x 10 milligram tube	20 milligrams
GLUCAGON (IM) 1 milligram per vial	500 micrograms	NONE	N/A	0.5 vial	500 micrograms
GLUCOSE 10% (IV) 50 grams in 500 ml	4 grams glucose	4 grams glucose	5 minutes	40 ml	120 ml (12 g glucose)
GLUCOSE 40% ORAL GEL (Buccal) 10 grams in 25 grams of gel	10 grams	10 grams	5 minutes	1 tube	2 tubes/20 grams
HYDROCORTISONE (IV/IO/IM) 100 milligrams in 1 ml	100 milligrams	NONE	N/A	1 ml	100 milligrams

Quick Reference Table — 6 YEARS — Page for Age

DRUG	INITIAL DOSE	REPEAT DOSE	DOSE INTERVAL	VOLUME	MAX DOSE
HYDROCORTISONE (IV/IO/IM) 100 milligrams in 2 ml	100 milligrams	NONE	N/A	2 ml	100 milligrams
IBUPROFEN (Oral) 100 milligrams in 5 ml	150 milligrams	150 milligrams	8 hours	7.5 ml	450 milligrams per 24 hours
IPRATROPIUM BROMIDE (Neb) 250 micrograms in 1 ml	250 micrograms	NONE	N/A	1 ml	250 micrograms
IPRATROPIUM BROMIDE (Neb) 500 micrograms in 2 ml	250 micrograms	NONE	N/A	1 ml	250 micrograms
MIDAZOLAM** (Buccal) 5 milligrams in 1 ml	7.5 milligrams	7.5 milligrams	10 mins	1.5 ml pre-filled syringe	15 milligrams
MORPHINE SULFATE (IV/IO) 10 milligrams in 10 ml	2 milligrams	2 milligrams	5 minutes	2 ml	4 milligrams
MORPHINE SULFATE (Oral) 10 milligrams in 5 ml	4 milligrams	NONE	N/A	2 ml	4 milligrams

**Give the dose as prescribed in the child's individual treatment plan/Epilepsy Passport (the dosages described above reflect the recommended dosages for a child of this age).

Quick Reference Table — 6 YEARS — Page for Age

DRUG	INITIAL DOSE	REPEAT DOSE	DOSE INTERVAL	VOLUME	MAX DOSE
NALOXONE (IV/IO) 400 micrograms in 1 ml	2,000 micrograms	Seek advice	N/A	5 ml	2,000 micrograms
NALOXONE (IM) 400 micrograms in 1 ml	400 micrograms	400 micrograms	3 minutes	1 ml	2,000 micrograms
ONDANSETRON (IV/IO/IM) 2 milligrams in 1 ml	2 milligrams	NONE	N/A	1 ml	2 milligrams
PARACETAMOL - SIX PLUS SUSPENSION (Oral) 250 milligrams in 5 ml	250 milligrams	250 milligrams	4–6 hours	5 ml	1 gram in 24 hours
PARACETAMOL (IV infusion/IO) 10 milligrams in 1 ml	300 milligrams	300 milligrams	4–6 hours	30 ml	1.2 grams in 24 hours
SALBUTAMOL (Neb) 2.5 milligrams in 2.5 ml	5 milligrams	5 milligrams	5 minutes	5 ml	No limit
SALBUTAMOL (Neb) 5 milligrams in 2.5 ml	5 milligrams	5 milligrams	5 minutes	2.5 ml	No limit
TRANEXAMIC ACID (IV) 100 mg/ml	300 mg	NONE	N/A	3 ml	300 mg

321

7 YEARS

Page for Age

Vital Signs

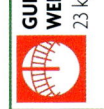

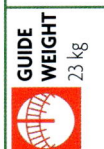

GUIDE WEIGHT	HEART RATE	RESPIRATION RATE	SYSTOLIC BLOOD PRESSURE
23 kg	80–120	20–25	90–110

Airway Size by Type

OROPHARYNGEAL AIRWAY	LARYNGEAL MASK	I-GEL AIRWAY	ENDOTRACHEAL TUBE
1 OR 2	2.5	2	Diameter: **6 mm**; Length: **16 cm**

Defibrillation – Cardiac Arrest

MANUAL	AUTOMATED EXTERNAL DEFIBRILLATOR
100 Joules	A standard AED (either with paediatric attenuation pads or else in paediatric mode) can be used. If paediatric pads are not available, standard adult pads can be used (but must not overlap).

Intravascular Fluid

FLUID	INITIAL DOSE	REPEAT DOSE	DOSE INTERVAL	VOLUME	MAX DOSE
Sodium Chloride (5 ml/kg) 0.9% (IV/IO)	115 ml	115 ml	PRN	115 ml	920 ml
Sodium Chloride (10 ml/kg) 0.9% (IV/IO)	230 ml	230 ml	PRN	230 ml	920 ml
Sodium Chloride (20 ml/kg) 0.9% (IV/IO)	460 ml	460 ml	PRN	460 ml	920 ml

7 YEARS — Page for Age

Cardiac Arrest

DRUG	INITIAL DOSE	REPEAT DOSE	DOSE INTERVAL	VOLUME	MAX DOSE
ADRENALINE **Cardiac Arrest** (IV/IO) 1 milligram in 10 ml (1:10,000)	230 micrograms	230 micrograms	3–5 minutes	2.3 ml	No limit
AMIODARONE **Cardiac Arrest** (IV/IO) 300 milligrams in 10 ml	120 milligrams (After 3rd shock)	120 milligrams	After 5th shock	4 ml	240 milligrams

Quick Reference Table

7 YEARS

Page for Age

DRUG	INITIAL DOSE	REPEAT DOSE	DOSE INTERVAL	VOLUME	MAX DOSE
ACTIVATED CHARCOAL* (Oral) 50 grams in 250 ml	25 g	25 g	N/A	125 ml	50 grams
ADRENALINE - ANAPHYLAXIS/ASTHMA (IM) 1 milligram in 1 ml (1:1,000)	300 micrograms	300 micrograms	5 minutes	0.3 ml	No limit
BENZYLPENICILLIN (IV/IO) 600 milligrams dissolved in 10 ml water for injection	600 milligrams	NONE	N/A	10 ml	600 milligrams
BENZYLPENICILLIN (IM) 600 milligrams dissolved in 2 ml water for injection	600 milligrams	NONE	N/A	2 ml	600 milligrams
CHLORPHENAMINE (IV/IO/IM) 10 milligrams in 1 ml	5 milligrams	NONE	N/A	0.5 ml	5 milligrams
CHLORPHENAMINE Oral (tablet) 4 milligrams per tablet	2 milligrams	NONE	N/A	½ of one tablet	2 milligrams
CHLORPHENAMINE Oral (solution) 2 milligrams in 5 ml	2 milligrams	NONE	N/A	5 ml	2 milligrams

*If a large quantity of poison has been ingested, and where there is a risk to life, encourage the child to drink the full dose.

Quick Reference Table

7 YEARS — Page for Age

DRUG	INITIAL DOSE	REPEAT DOSE	DOSE INTERVAL	VOLUME	MAX DOSE
DEXAMETHASONE Oral (solution) 2 milligrams in 5 ml	4 milligrams	NONE	N/A	10 ml	4 milligrams
DEXAMETHASONE Oral (tablet) 2 milligrams per tablet	4 milligrams	NONE	N/A	2 tablets	4 milligrams
DIAZEPAM (IV/IO) 10 milligrams in 2 ml	7 milligrams	7 milligrams	10 minutes	1.4 ml	14 milligrams
DIAZEPAM (Rectal) 10 milligrams in 2.5 ml	10 milligrams	10 milligrams	10 minutes	1 x 10 milligram tube	20 milligrams
GLUCAGON (IM) 1 milligram per vial	500 micrograms	NONE	N/A	0.5 vial	500 micrograms
GLUCOSE 10% (IV) 50 grams in 500 ml	5 grams glucose	5 grams glucose	5 minutes	50 ml	150 ml (15 g glucose)
GLUCOSE 40% ORAL GEL (Buccal) 10 grams in 25 grams of gel	10 grams	10 grams	5 minutes	1 tube	2 tubes /20 grams
HYDROCORTISONE (IV/IO/IM) 100 milligrams in 1 ml	100 milligrams	NONE	N/A	1 ml	100 milligrams

Quick Reference Table — 7 YEARS — Page for Age

DRUG	INITIAL DOSE	REPEAT DOSE	DOSE INTERVAL	VOLUME	MAX DOSE
HYDROCORTISONE (IV/IO/IM) 100 milligrams in 2 ml	100 milligrams	NONE	N/A	2 ml	100 milligrams
IBUPROFEN (Oral) 100 milligrams in 5 ml	200 milligrams	200 milligrams	8 hours	10 ml	600 milligrams per 24 hours
IPRATROPIUM BROMIDE (Neb) 250 micrograms in 1 ml	250 micrograms	NONE	N/A	1 ml	250 micrograms
IPRATROPIUM BROMIDE (Neb) 500 micrograms in 2 ml	250 micrograms	NONE	N/A	1 ml	250 micrograms
MIDAZOLAM** (Buccal) 5 milligrams in 1 ml	7.5 milligrams	7.5 milligrams	10 mins	1.5 ml pre-filled syringe	15 milligrams
MORPHINE SULFATE (IV/IO) 10 milligrams in 10 ml	2.5 milligrams	2.5 milligrams	5 minutes	2.5 ml	5 milligrams
MORPHINE SULFATE (Oral) 10 milligrams in 5 ml	5 milligrams	NONE	N/A	2.5 ml	5 milligrams

**Give the dose as prescribed in the child's individual treatment plan/Epilepsy Passport (the dosages described above reflect the recommended dosages for a child of this age).

Quick Reference Table

7 YEARS
Page for Age

DRUG	INITIAL DOSE	REPEAT DOSE	DOSE INTERVAL	VOLUME	MAX DOSE
NALOXONE (IV/IO) 400 micrograms in 1 ml	2,000 micrograms	Seek advice	N/A	5 ml	2,000 micrograms
NALOXONE (IM) 400 micrograms in 1 ml	400 micrograms	400 micrograms	3 minutes	1 ml	2,000 micrograms
ONDANSETRON (IV/IO/IM) 2 milligrams in 1 ml	2.5 milligrams	NONE	N/A	1.3 ml	2.5 milligrams
PARACETAMOL PLUS SUSPENSION (Oral) 250 milligrams in 5 ml	250 milligrams	250 milligrams	4-6 hours	5 ml	1 gram in 24 hours
PARACETAMOL (IV infusion/IO) 10 milligrams in 1 ml	350 milligrams	350 milligrams	4-6 hours	35 ml	1.4 grams in 24 hours
SALBUTAMOL (Neb) 2.5 milligrams in 2.5 ml	5 milligrams	5 milligrams	5 minutes	5 ml	No limit
SALBUTAMOL (Neb) 5 milligrams in 2.5 ml	5 milligrams	5 milligrams	5 minutes	2.5 ml	No limit
TRANEXAMIC ACID (IV) 100 mg/ml	350 mg	NONE	N/A	3.5 ml	350 mg

8 YEARS

Page for Age

Vital Signs

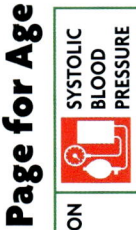

GUIDE WEIGHT	HEART RATE	RESPIRATION RATE	SYSTOLIC BLOOD PRESSURE
26 kg	80–120	20–25	90–110

Airway Size by Type

OROPHARYNGEAL AIRWAY	LARYNGEAL MASK	I-GEL AIRWAY	ENDOTRACHEAL TUBE
1 OR 2	2.5	2.5	Diameter: **6.5 mm**; Length: **17 cm**

Defibrillation – Cardiac Arrest

MANUAL	AUTOMATED EXTERNAL DEFIBRILLATOR
100 Joules	A standard AED (either with paediatric attenuation pads or else in paediatric mode) can be used. If paediatric pads are not available, standard adult pads can be used (but must not overlap).

Intravascular Fluid

FLUID	INITIAL DOSE	REPEAT DOSE	DOSE INTERVAL	VOLUME	MAX DOSE
Sodium Chloride (5 ml/kg) (IV/IO) 0.9%	130 ml	130 ml	PRN	130 ml	1,000 ml
Sodium Chloride (10 ml/kg) (IV/IO) 0.9%	250 ml	250 ml	PRN	250 ml	1,000 ml
Sodium Chloride (20 ml/kg) (IV/IO) 0.9%	500 ml	500 ml	PRN	500 ml	1,000 ml

Cardiac Arrest

8 YEARS Page for Age

DRUG	INITIAL DOSE	REPEAT DOSE	DOSE INTERVAL	VOLUME	MAX DOSE
ADRENALINE **Cardiac Arrest** (IV/IO) 1 milligram in 10 ml (1:10,000)	260 micrograms	260 micrograms	3–5 minutes	2.6 ml	No limit
AMIODARONE **Cardiac Arrest** (IV/IO) 300 milligrams in 10 ml	130 milligrams (After 3rd shock)	130 milligrams	After 5th shock	43 ml	260 milligrams

Quick Reference Table — 8 YEARS — Page for Age

DRUG	INITIAL DOSE	REPEAT DOSE	DOSE INTERVAL	VOLUME	MAX DOSE
ACTIVATED CHARCOAL* (Oral) 50 grams in 250 ml	25 g	25 g	N/A	125 ml	50 grams
ADRENALINE - ANAPHYLAXIS/ASTHMA (IM) 1 milligram in 1 ml (1:1,000)	300 micrograms	300 micrograms	5 minutes	0.3 ml	No limit
BENZYLPENICILLIN (IV/IO) 600 milligrams dissolved in 10 ml water for injection	600 milligrams	NONE	N/A	10 ml	600 milligrams
BENZYLPENICILLIN (IM) 600 milligrams dissolved in 2 ml water for injection	600 milligrams	NONE	N/A	2 ml	600 milligrams
CHLORPHENAMINE (IV/IO/IM) 10 milligrams in 1 ml	5 milligrams	NONE	N/A	0.5 ml	5 milligrams
CHLORPHENAMINE Oral (tablet) 4 milligrams per tablet	2 milligrams	NONE	N/A	½ of one tablet	2 milligrams
CHLORPHENAMINE Oral (solution) 2 milligrams in 5 ml	2 milligrams	NONE	N/A	5 ml	2 milligrams

*If a large quantity of poison has been ingested, and where there is a risk to life, encourage the child to drink the full dose.

Quick Reference Table

8 YEARS Page for Age

DRUG	INITIAL DOSE	REPEAT DOSE	DOSE INTERVAL	VOLUME	MAX DOSE
DEXAMETHASONE Oral (solution) 2 milligrams in 5 ml		NONE	N/A	10 ml	4 milligrams
DEXAMETHASONE Oral (tablet) 2 milligrams per tablet		NONE	N/A	2 tablets	
DIAZEPAM (IV/IO) 10 milligrams in 2 ml	8 milligrams	8 milligrams	10 minutes	1.6 ml	16 milligrams
DIAZEPAM (Rectal) 10 milligrams in 2.5 ml		10 milligrams	10 minutes	1 x 10 milligram tube	
GLUCAGON (IM) 1 milligram per vial	1 milligram	NONE	N/A	1 vial	1 milligram
GLUCOSE 10% (IV) 50 grams in 500 ml	5 grams glucose	5 grams glucose	5 minutes	50 ml	150 ml (15 g glucose)
GLUCOSE 40% ORAL GEL (buccal) 10 grams in 25 grams of gel		10 grams	5 minutes	1 tube	
HYDROCORTISONE (IV/IO/IM) 100 milligrams in 1 ml		NONE	N/A	1 ml	

Quick Reference Table — 8 YEARS — Page for Age

DRUG	INITIAL DOSE	REPEAT DOSE	DOSE INTERVAL	VOLUME	MAX DOSE
HYDROCORTISONE (IV/IO/IM) 100 milligrams in 2 ml	100 milligrams	NONE	N/A	2 ml	100 milligrams
IBUPROFEN (Oral) 100 milligrams in 5 ml	200 milligrams	200 milligrams	8 hours	10 ml	600 milligrams per 24 hours
IPRATROPIUM BROMIDE (Neb) 250 micrograms in 1 ml	250 micrograms	NONE	N/A	1 ml	250 micrograms
IPRATROPIUM BROMIDE (Neb) 500 micrograms in 2 ml	250 micrograms	NONE	N/A	1 ml	250 micrograms
MIDAZOLAM** (Buccal) 5 milligrams in 1 ml	7.5 milligrams	7.5 milligrams	10 mins	1.5 ml pre-filled syringe	15 milligrams
MORPHINE SULFATE (IV/IO) 10 milligrams in 10 ml	2.5 milligrams	2.5 milligrams	5 minutes	2.5 ml	5 milligrams
MORPHINE SULFATE (Oral) 10 milligrams in 5 ml	5 milligrams	NONE	N/A	2.5 ml	5 milligrams
NALOXONE (IV/IO) 400 micrograms in 1 ml	2,000 micrograms	Seek advice	N/A	5 ml	2,000 micrograms

**Give the dose as prescribed in the child's individual treatment plan/Epilepsy Passport (the dosages described above reflect the recommended dosages for a child of this age).

Quick Reference Table — 8 YEARS — Page for Age

DRUG	INITIAL DOSE	REPEAT DOSE	DOSE INTERVAL	VOLUME	MAX DOSE
NALOXONE (IM) 400 micrograms in 1 ml	400 micrograms	400 micrograms	3 minutes	1 ml	2,000 micrograms
ONDANSETRON (IV/IO/IM) 2 milligrams in 1 ml	2.5 milligrams	NONE	N/A	1.3 ml	2.5 milligrams
PARACETAMOL - SIX PLUS SUSPENSION (Oral) 250 milligrams in 5 ml	375 milligrams	375 milligrams	4–6 hours	7.5 ml	1.5 grams in 24 hours
PARACETAMOL (IV infusion/IO) 10 milligrams in 1 ml	400 milligrams	400 milligrams	4–6 hours	40 ml	1.6 grams in 24 hours
SALBUTAMOL (Neb) 2.5 milligrams in 2.5 ml	5 milligrams	5 milligrams	5 minutes	5 ml	No limit
SALBUTAMOL (Neb) 5 milligrams in 2.5 ml	5 milligrams	5 milligrams	5 minutes	2.5 ml	No limit
TRANEXAMIC ACID (IV) 100 mg/ml	400 mg	NONE	N/A	4 ml	400 mg

333

9 YEARS — Page for Age

Vital Signs

GUIDE WEIGHT	HEART RATE	RESPIRATION RATE	SYSTOLIC BLOOD PRESSURE
29 kg	80–120	20–25	90–110

Airway Size by Type

OROPHARYNGEAL AIRWAY	LARYNGEAL MASK	I-GEL AIRWAY	ENDOTRACHEAL TUBE
1 OR 2	2.5	2.5	Diameter: **6.5 mm**; Length: **17 cm**

Defibrillation – Cardiac Arrest

MANUAL	AUTOMATED EXTERNAL DEFIBRILLATOR
120 Joules	A standard AED can be used (without the need for paediatric attenuation pads).

Intravascular Fluid

FLUID	INITIAL DOSE	REPEAT DOSE	DOSE INTERVAL	VOLUME	MAX DOSE
Sodium Chloride (5 ml/kg) 0.9% (IV/IO)	145 ml	145 ml	PRN	145 ml	1,000 ml
Sodium Chloride (10 ml/kg) 0.9% (IV/IO)	290 ml	290 ml	PRN	290 ml	1,000 ml
Sodium Chloride (20 ml/kg) 0.9% (IV/IO)	500 ml	500 ml	PRN	500 ml	1,000 ml

Cardiac Arrest

9 YEARS — Page for Age

DRUG	INITIAL DOSE	REPEAT DOSE	DOSE INTERVAL	VOLUME	MAX DOSE
ADRENALINE **Cardiac Arrest** (IV/IO) 1 milligram in 10 ml (1:10,000)	300 micrograms	300 micrograms	3–5 minutes	3 ml	No limit
AMIODARONE **Cardiac Arrest** (IV/IO) 300 milligrams in 10 ml	150 milligrams (After 3rd shock)	150 milligrams	After 5th shock	5 ml	300 milligrams

Quick Reference Table — 9 YEARS — Page for Age

DRUG	INITIAL DOSE	REPEAT DOSE	DOSE INTERVAL	VOLUME	MAX DOSE
ACTIVATED CHARCOAL* (Oral) 50 grams in 250 ml	25 g	25 g	N/A	125 ml	50 grams
ADRENALINE - ANAPHYLAXIS/ASTHMA (IM) 1 milligram in 1 ml (1:1,000)	300 micrograms	300 micrograms	5 minutes	0.3 ml	No limit
BENZYLPENICILLIN (IV/IO) 600 milligrams dissolved in 10 ml water for injection	600 milligrams	NONE	N/A	10 ml	600 milligrams
BENZYLPENICILLIN (IM) 600 milligrams dissolved in 2 ml water for injection	600 milligrams	NONE	N/A	2 ml	600 milligrams
CHLORPHENAMINE (IV/IO/IM) 10 milligrams in 1 ml	5 milligrams	NONE	N/A	0.5 ml	5 milligrams
CHLORPHENAMINE Oral (tablet) 4 milligrams per tablet	2 milligrams	NONE	N/A	½ of one tablet	2 milligrams

*If a large quantity of poison has been ingested, and where there is a risk to life, encourage the child to drink the full dose.

Quick Reference Table

9 YEARS — Page for Age

DRUG	INITIAL DOSE	REPEAT DOSE	DOSE INTERVAL	VOLUME	MAX DOSE
CHLORPHENAMINE Oral (solution) 2 milligrams in 5 ml	2 milligrams	NONE	N/A	5 ml	2 milligrams
DEXAMETHASONE Oral (solution) 2 milligrams in 5 ml	6 milligrams	NONE	N/A	15 ml	6 milligrams
DEXAMETHASONE Oral (tablet) 2 milligrams per tablet	6 milligrams	NONE	N/A	3 tablets	6 milligrams
DIAZEPAM (IV/IO) 10 milligrams in 2 ml	9 milligrams	9 milligrams	10 minutes	1.8 ml	18 milligrams
DIAZEPAM (Rectal) 10 milligrams in 2.5 ml	10 milligrams	10 milligrams	10 minutes	1 x 10 milligram tube	20 milligrams
GLUCAGON (IM) 1 milligram per vial	1 milligram	NONE	N/A	1 vial	1 milligram
GLUCOSE 10% (IV) 50 grams in 500 ml	6 grams glucose	6 grams glucose	5 minutes	60 ml	180 ml (18 g glucose)
GLUCOSE 40% ORAL GEL (Buccal) 10 grams in 25 grams of gel	10 grams	10 grams	5 minutes	1 tube	2 tubes / 20 grams

Quick Reference Table — 9 YEARS — Page for Age

DRUG	INITIAL DOSE	REPEAT DOSE	DOSE INTERVAL	VOLUME	MAX DOSE
HYDROCORTISONE (IV/IO/IM) 100 milligrams in 1 ml	100 milligrams	NONE	N/A	1 ml	100 milligrams
HYDROCORTISONE (IV/IO/IM) 100 milligrams in 2 ml	100 milligrams	NONE	N/A	2 ml	100 milligrams
IBUPROFEN (Oral) 100 milligrams in 5 ml	200 milligrams	200 milligrams	8 hours	10 ml	600 milligrams per 24 hours
IPRATROPIUM BROMIDE (Neb) 250 micrograms in 1 ml	250 micrograms	NONE	N/A	1 ml	250 micrograms
IPRATROPIUM BROMIDE (Neb) 500 micrograms in 2 ml	250 micrograms	NONE	N/A	1 ml	250 micrograms
MIDAZOLAM** (Buccal) 5 milligrams in 1 ml	7.5 milligrams	7.5 milligrams	10 mins	1.5 ml pre-filled syringe	15 milligrams
MORPHINE SULFATE (IV/IO) 10 milligrams in 10 ml	3 milligrams	3 milligrams	5 minutes	3 ml	6 milligrams

**Give the dose as prescribed in the child's individual treatment plan/Epilepsy Passport (the dosages described above reflect the recommended dosages for a child of this age).

Quick Reference Table

9 YEARS Page for Age

DRUG	INITIAL DOSE	REPEAT DOSE	DOSE INTERVAL	VOLUME	MAX DOSE
MORPHINE SULFATE (Oral) 10 milligrams in 5 ml	6 milligrams	NONE	N/A	3 ml	6 milligrams
NALOXONE (IV/IO) 400 micrograms in 1 ml	2,000 micrograms	Seek advice	N/A	5 ml	2,000 micrograms
NALOXONE (IM) 400 micrograms in 1 ml	400 micrograms	400 micrograms	3 minutes	1 ml	2,000 micrograms
ONDANSETRON (IV/IO/IM) 2 milligrams in 1 ml	3 milligrams	NONE	N/A	1.5 ml	3 milligrams
PARACETAMOL - SIX PLUS SUSPENSION (Oral) 250 milligrams in 5 ml	375 milligrams	375 milligrams	4–6 hours	7.5 ml	1.5 grams in 24 hours
PARACETAMOL (IV infusion/IO) 10 milligrams in 1 ml	450 milligrams	450 milligrams	4–6 hours	45 ml	1.8 grams in 24 hours
SALBUTAMOL (Neb) 2.5 milligrams 2.5 ml	5 milligrams	5 milligrams	5 minutes	5 ml	No limit
SALBUTAMOL (Neb) 5 milligrams in 2.5 ml	5 milligrams	5 milligrams	5 minutes	2.5 ml	No limit
TRANEXAMIC ACID (IV) 100 mg/ml	450 mg	NONE	N/A	4.5 ml	450 mg

10 YEARS — Page for Age

Vital Signs

GUIDE WEIGHT	HEART RATE	RESPIRATION RATE	SYSTOLIC BLOOD PRESSURE
32 kg	80–120	20–25	90–110

Airway Size by Type

OROPHARYNGEAL AIRWAY	LARYNGEAL MASK	I-GEL AIRWAY	ENDOTRACHEAL TUBE
2 OR 3	3	2.5 OR 3	Diameter: **7 mm**; Length: **18 cm**

Defibrillation – Cardiac Arrest

MANUAL	AUTOMATED EXTERNAL DEFIBRILLATOR
130 Joules	A standard AED can be used (without the need for paediatric attenuation pads).

Intravascular Fluid

FLUID	INITIAL DOSE	REPEAT DOSE	DOSE INTERVAL	VOLUME	MAX DOSE
Sodium Chloride (5 ml/kg) (IV/IO) 0.9%	160 ml	160 ml	PRN	160 ml	1,000 ml
Sodium Chloride (10 ml/kg) (IV/IO) 0.9%	320 ml	320 ml	PRN	320 ml	1,000 ml
Sodium Chloride (20 ml/kg) (IV/IO) 0.9%	500 ml	500 ml	PRN	500 ml	1,000 ml

Cardiac Arrest

10 YEARS — Page for Age

DRUG	INITIAL DOSE	REPEAT DOSE	DOSE INTERVAL	VOLUME	MAX DOSE
ADRENALINE **Cardiac Arrest** (IV/IO) 1 milligram in 10 ml (1:10,000)	320 micrograms	320 micrograms	3–5 minutes	3.2 ml	No limit
AMIODARONE **Cardiac Arrest** (IV/IO) 300 milligrams in 10 ml	160 milligrams (After 3rd shock)	160 milligrams	After 5th shock	5.3 ml	320 milligrams

Quick Reference Table — 10 YEARS — Page for Age

DRUG	INITIAL DOSE	REPEAT DOSE	DOSE INTERVAL	VOLUME	MAX DOSE
ACTIVATED CHARCOAL* (Oral) 50 grams in 250 ml	25 g	25 g	N/A	125 ml	50 grams
ADRENALINE - ANAPHYLAXIS/ASTHMA (IM) 1 milligram in 1 ml (1:1,000)	300 micrograms	300 micrograms	5 minutes	0.3 ml	No limit
BENZYLPENICILLIN (IV/IO) 1.2 grams dissolved in 20 ml water for injection	1.2 grams	NONE	N/A	20 ml	1.2 grams
BENZYLPENICILLIN (IM) 1.2 grams dissolved in 4 ml water for injection	1.2 grams	NONE	N/A	4 ml	1.2 grams
CHLORPHENAMINE (IV/IO/IM) 10 milligrams in 1 ml	5 milligrams	NONE	N/A	0.5 ml	5 milligrams
CHLORPHENAMINE Oral (tablet) 4 milligrams per tablet	2 milligrams	NONE	N/A	½ of one tablet	2 milligrams
CHLORPHENAMINE Oral (solution) 2 milligrams in 5 ml	2 milligrams	NONE	N/A	5 ml	2 milligrams

*If a large quantity of poison has been ingested, and where there is a risk to life, encourage the child to drink the full dose.

Quick Reference Table

10 YEARS — Page for Age

DRUG	INITIAL DOSE	REPEAT DOSE	DOSE INTERVAL	VOLUME	MAX DOSE
DEXAMETHASONE Oral (solution) 2 milligrams in 5 ml	6 milligrams	NONE	N/A	15 ml	6 milligrams
DEXAMETHASONE Oral (tablet) 2 milligrams per tablet	6 milligrams	NONE	N/A	3 tablets	6 milligrams
DIAZEPAM (IV/IO) 10 milligrams in 2 ml	10 milligrams	10 milligrams	10 minutes	2 ml	20 milligrams
DIAZEPAM (Rectal) 10 milligrams in 2.5 ml	10 milligrams	10 milligrams	10 minutes	1 x 10 milligram tube	20 milligrams
GLUCAGON (IM) 1 milligram per vial	1 milligram	NONE	N/A	1 vial	1 milligram
GLUCOSE 10% (IV) 50 grams in 500 ml	6.5 grams glucose	6.5 grams glucose	5 minutes	65 ml	195 ml (19.5 g glucose)
GLUCOSE 40% ORAL GEL (Buccal) 10 grams in 25 grams of gel	10 grams	10 grams	5 minutes	1 tube	2 tubes/20 grams
HYDROCORTISONE (IV/IO/IM) 100 milligrams in 1 ml	100 milligrams	NONE	N/A	1 ml	100 milligrams

RESUS PAED GENERAL MEDICAL TRAUMA SP SITU MATERNITY MEDS **PAGE AGE** 343

Quick Reference Table — 10 YEARS — Page for Age

DRUG	INITIAL DOSE	REPEAT DOSE	DOSE INTERVAL	VOLUME	MAX DOSE
HYDROCORTISONE (IV/IO/IM) 100 milligrams in 2 ml	100 milligrams	NONE	N/A	2 ml	100 milligrams
IBUPROFEN (Oral) 100 milligrams in 5 ml	300 milligrams	300 milligrams	8 hours	15 ml	900 milligrams per 24 hours
IPRATROPIUM BROMIDE (Neb) 500 micrograms in 2 ml	250 micrograms	NONE	N/A	1 ml	250 micrograms
IPRATROPIUM BROMIDE (Neb) 250 micrograms in 1 ml	250 micrograms	NONE	N/A	1 ml	250 micrograms
MIDAZOLAM** (Buccal) 5 milligrams in 1 ml	10 milligrams	10 milligrams	10 mins	2 ml pre-filled syringe	20 milligrams
MORPHINE SULFATE (IV/IO) 10 milligrams in 10 ml	3 milligrams	3 milligrams	5 minutes	3 ml	6 milligrams
MORPHINE SULFATE (Oral) 10 milligrams in 5 ml	6 milligrams	NONE	N/A	3 ml	6 milligrams

**Give the dose as prescribed in the child's individual treatment plan/Epilepsy Passport (the dosages described above reflect the recommended dosages for a child of this age).

Quick Reference Table

10 YEARS Page for Age

DRUG	INITIAL DOSE	REPEAT DOSE	DOSE INTERVAL	VOLUME	MAX DOSE
NALOXONE (IV/IO) 400 micrograms in 1 ml	2,000 micrograms	Seek advice	N/A	5 ml	2,000 micrograms
NALOXONE (IM) 400 micrograms in 1 ml	400 micrograms	400 micrograms	3 minutes	1 ml	2,000 micrograms
ONDANSETRON (IV/IO/IM) 2 milligrams in 1 ml	3 milligrams	NONE	N/A	1.5 ml	3 milligrams
PARACETAMOL - SIX PLUS SUSPENSION (Oral) 250 milligrams in 5 ml	500 milligrams	500 milligrams	4-6 hours	10 ml	2 grams in 24 hours
PARACETAMOL (IV infusion/IO) 10 milligrams in 1 ml	500 milligrams	500 milligrams	4-6 hours	50 ml	2 grams in 24 hours
SALBUTAMOL (Neb) 2.5 milligrams in 2.5 ml	5 milligrams	5 milligrams	5 minutes	5 ml	No limit
SALBUTAMOL (Neb) 5 milligrams in 2.5 ml	5 milligrams	5 milligrams	5 minutes	2.5 ml	No limit
TRANEXAMIC ACID (IV) 100 mg/ml	500 mg	NONE	N/A	5 ml	500 mg

345

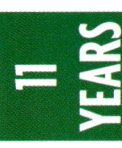

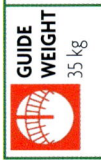

Page for Age

11 YEARS

Vital Signs

GUIDE WEIGHT	HEART RATE	RESPIRATION RATE	SYSTOLIC BLOOD PRESSURE
35 kg	80–120	20–25	90–110

Airway Size by Type

OROPHARYNGEAL AIRWAY	LARYNGEAL MASK	I-GEL AIRWAY	ENDOTRACHEAL TUBE
2 OR 3	3	2.5 OR 3	Diameter: **7 mm**; Length: **18 cm**

Defibrillation – Cardiac Arrest

MANUAL	AUTOMATED EXTERNAL DEFIBRILLATOR
140 Joules	A standard AED can be used (without the need for paediatric attenuation pads).

Intravascular Fluid

FLUID	INITIAL DOSE	REPEAT DOSE	DOSE INTERVAL	VOLUME	MAX DOSE
Sodium Chloride (5 ml/kg) (IV/IO) 0.9%	175 ml	175 ml	PRN	175 ml	1,000 ml
Sodium Chloride (10 ml/kg) (IV/IO) 0.9%	350 ml	350 ml	PRN	350 ml	1,000 ml
Sodium Chloride (20 ml/kg) (IV/IO) 0.9%	500 ml	500 ml	PRN	500 ml	1,000 ml

Cardiac Arrest

11 YEARS — Page for Age

DRUG	INITIAL DOSE	REPEAT DOSE	DOSE INTERVAL	VOLUME	MAX DOSE
ADRENALINE **Cardiac Arrest** (IV/IO) 1 milligram in 10 ml (1:10,000)	350 micrograms	350 micrograms	3–5 minutes	3.5 ml	No limit
AMIODARONE **Cardiac Arrest** (IV/IO) 300 milligrams in 10 ml	180 milligrams (After 3rd shock)	180 milligrams	After 5th shock	6 ml	360 milligrams

347

Quick Reference Table — 11 YEARS — Page for Age

DRUG	INITIAL DOSE	REPEAT DOSE	DOSE INTERVAL	VOLUME	MAX DOSE
ACTIVATED CHARCOAL* (Oral) 50 grams in 250 ml	25 g	25 g	N/A	125 ml	50 grams
ADRENALINE - ANAPHYLAXIS/ASTHMA (IM) 1 milligram in 1 ml (1:1,000)	300 micrograms	300 micrograms	5 minutes	0.3 ml	No limit
BENZYLPENICILLIN (IV/IO) 1.2 grams dissolved in 20 ml water for injection	1.2 grams	NONE	N/A	20 ml	1.2 grams
BENZYLPENICILLIN (IM) 1.2 grams dissolved in 4 ml water for injection	1.2 grams	NONE	N/A	4 ml	1.2 grams
CHLORPHENAMINE (IV/IO/IM) 10 milligrams in 1 ml	5 milligrams	NONE	N/A	0.5 ml	5 milligrams
CHLORPHENAMINE Oral (tablet) 4 milligrams per tablet	2 milligrams	NONE	N/A	½ of one tablet	2 milligrams
CHLORPHENAMINE Oral (solution) 2 milligrams in 5 ml	2 milligrams	NONE	N/A	5 ml	2 milligrams

*If a large quantity of poison has been ingested, and where there is a risk to life, encourage the child to drink the full dose.

Quick Reference Table

11 YEARS Page for Age

DRUG	INITIAL DOSE	REPEAT DOSE	DOSE INTERVAL	VOLUME	MAX DOSE
DEXAMETHASONE Oral (solution) 2 milligrams in 5 ml	6 milligrams	NONE	N/A	15 ml	6 milligrams
DEXAMETHASONE Oral (tablet) 2 milligrams per tablet	6 milligrams	NONE	N/A	3 tablets	6 milligrams
DIAZEPAM (IV/IO) 10 milligrams in 2 ml	10 milligrams	10 milligrams	10 minutes	2 ml	20 milligrams
DIAZEPAM (Rectal) 10 milligrams in 2.5 ml	10 milligrams	10 milligrams	10 minutes	1 x 10 milligram tube	20 milligrams
GLUCAGON (IM) 1 milligram per vial	1 milligram	NONE	N/A	1 vial	1 milligram
GLUCOSE 10% (IV) 50 grams in 500 ml	7 grams glucose	7 grams glucose	5 minutes	70 ml	210 ml (21g glucose)
GLUCOSE 40% ORAL GEL (Buccal) 10 grams in 25 grams of gel	10 grams	10 grams	5 minutes	1 tube	2 tubes/20 grams
HYDROCORTISONE (IV/IO/IM) 100 milligrams in 1 ml	100 milligrams	NONE	N/A	1 ml	100 milligrams

Quick Reference Table — 11 YEARS — Page for Age

DRUG	INITIAL DOSE	REPEAT DOSE	DOSE INTERVAL	VOLUME	MAX DOSE
HYDROCORTISONE (IV/IO/IM) 100 milligrams in 2 ml	100 milligrams	NONE	N/A	2 ml	100 milligrams
IBUPROFEN (Oral) 100 milligrams in 5 ml	300 milligrams	300 milligrams	8 hours	15 ml	900 milligrams per 24 hours
IPRATROPIUM BROMIDE (Neb) 250 micrograms in 1 ml	250 micrograms	NONE	N/A	1 ml	250 micrograms
IPRATROPIUM BROMIDE (Neb) 500 micrograms in 2 ml	250 micrograms	NONE	N/A	1 ml	250 micrograms
MIDAZOLAM** (Buccal) 5 milligrams in 1 ml	10 milligrams	10 milligrams	10 mins	2 ml pre-filled syringe	20 milligrams
MORPHINE SULFATE (IV/IO) 10 milligrams in 10 ml	3.5 milligrams	3.5 milligrams	5 minutes	3.5 ml	7 milligrams
MORPHINE SULFATE (Oral) 10 milligrams in 5 ml	7 milligrams	NONE	N/A	3.5 ml	7 milligrams

**Give the dose as prescribed in the child's individual treatment plan/Epilepsy Passport (the dosages described above reflect the recommended dosages for a child of this age).

Quick Reference Table

11 YEARS — Page for Age

DRUG	INITIAL DOSE	REPEAT DOSE	DOSE INTERVAL	VOLUME	MAX DOSE
NALOXONE (IV/IO) 400 micrograms in 1 ml	2,000 micrograms	Seek advice	N/A	5 ml	2,000 micrograms
NALOXONE (IM) 400 micrograms in 1 ml	400 micrograms	400 micrograms	3 minutes	1 ml	2,000 micrograms
ONDANSETRON (IV/IO/IM) 2 milligrams in 1 ml	3 milligrams	NONE	N/A	1.5 ml	3 milligrams
PARACETAMOL - SIX PLUS SUSPENSION (Oral) 250 milligrams in 5 ml	500 milligrams	500 milligrams	4–6 hours	10 ml	2 grams in 24 hours
PARACETAMOL (IV infusion/IO) 10 milligrams in 1 ml	500 milligrams	500 milligrams	4–6 hours	50 ml	2 grams in 24 hours
SALBUTAMOL (Neb) 5 milligrams in 2.5 ml	5 milligrams	5 milligrams	5 minutes	2.5 ml	No limit
SALBUTAMOL (Neb) 2.5 milligrams in 2.5 ml	5 milligrams	5 milligrams	5 minutes	5 ml	No limit
TRANEXAMIC ACID (IV) 100 mg/ml	500 mg	NONE	N/A	5 ml	500 mg

This page left intentionally blank for your notes

This page left intentionally blank for your notes